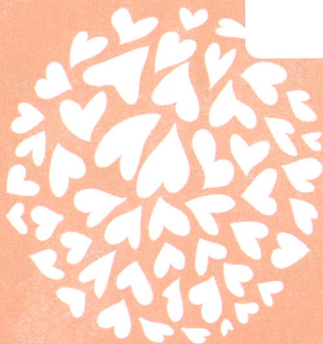

Beautiful You

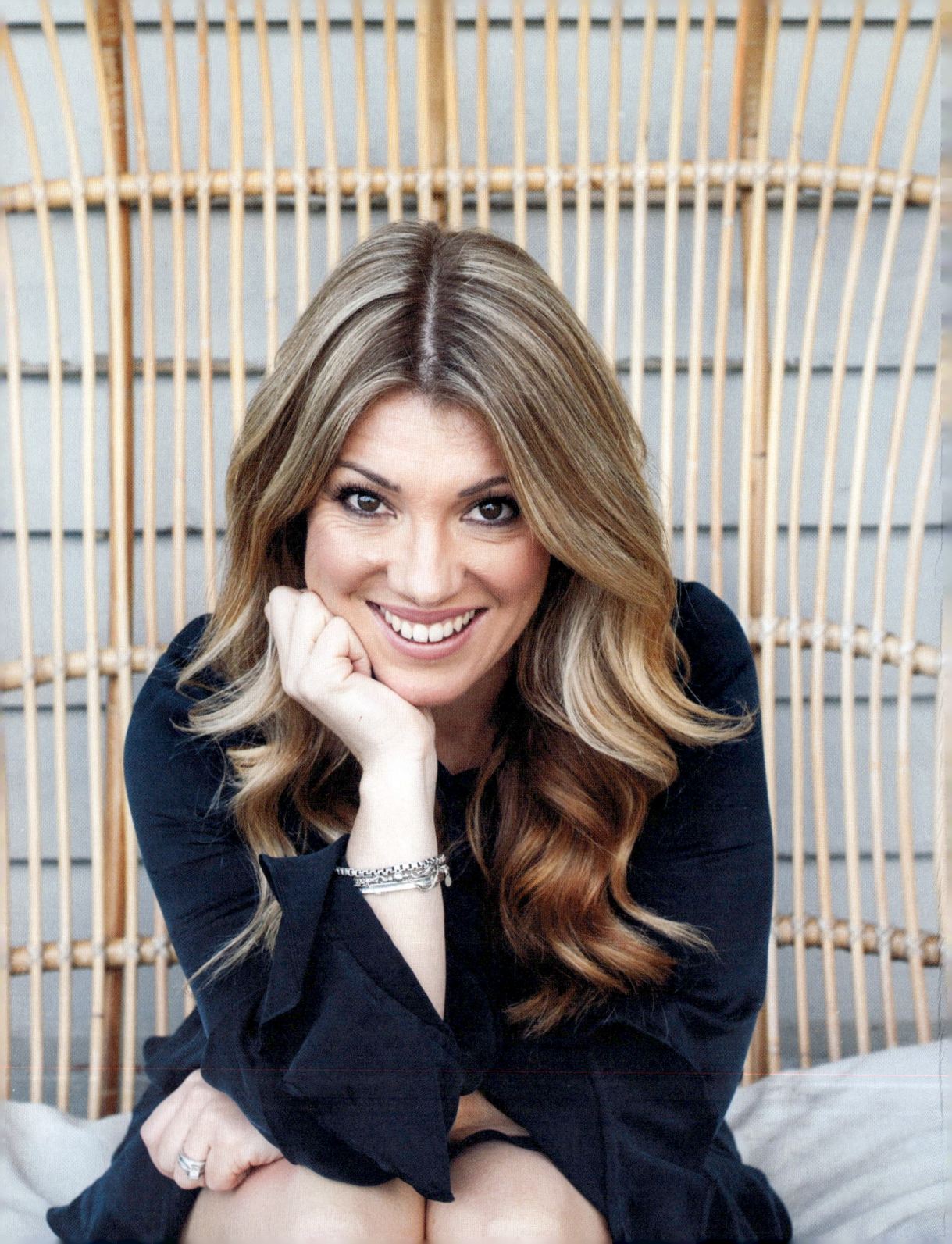

Beautiful You

Nat Kringoudis

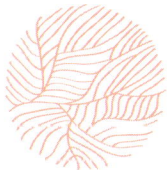

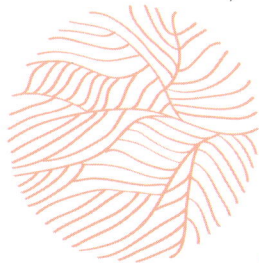

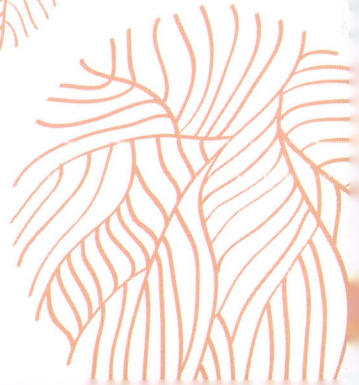

NON FICTION HQ

Contents

Foreword 7

Introduction 11

CHAPTER 1

Your hormones 18

The real secret to a happier, healthier you!

CHAPTER 2

Your mindset 52

Switching it on to grow and glow

CHAPTER 3

Your body changes 72

Playing detective – using your symptoms as your clues

CHAPTER 4

Hormone imbalances 92

What goes up can come down

CHAPTER 5

Your body challenges 146

Using symptoms to empower you

CHAPTER 6

Your options 162

Finding the answers within us

CHAPTER 7

Your wellbeing 178

Feeling good more often

CHAPTER 8

What's the deal, 'down there'? 192

I swear that rogue hair wasn't there yesterday!

CHAPTER 9

Your doctor 210

Only you know how you feel inside

CHAPTER 10

You are what you eat 222

Nobody wants to be a hotdog

CHAPTER 11

Your affirmations 272

You're a boss

Getting down to business – your 3-month program 283

Thanks 297

Index 300

IMPORTANT NOTE:

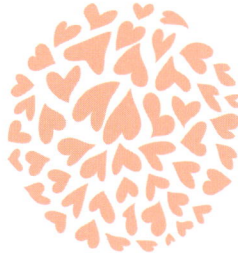

Foreword

On an early Friday morning in clinic I entered an exam room where I encountered a 13-year-old girl and her mother. The teenager was obviously distraught and her mother had a look of complete exhaustion. Over the course of the visit it was obvious that the young girl was having issues with her period, in the sense that she didn't want it, and it was embarrassing to her; she was having issues using tampons and didn't like the feel of pads. Her mother was helping her, but was becoming frustrated because her daughter couldn't get past the fact that this was a normal process. It occurred to me in that room years ago that young women in this century have become familiar with their reproductive areas, in the sense that they begin shaving and caring for the area, but they really aren't that comfortable with what is going on inside. I also saw that mothers, in this age of mobile phones and Google, are losing the battle with educating their young daughters on how the female reproductive system works.

The book you are holding is a treasure of information that not only will help mothers educate their daughters, but will give younger women a sense of empowerment and education that can make the unseen understandable and approachable. As parents – my first-born child is a daughter – we can find it difficult to educate and normalise certain aspects of life because we are pre-empted by text messages and YouTube videos, but we are also the primary educators of our children. Young girls reading this book will find information that is not only easy to understand but presented by Dr Natalie Kringoudis, who is internationally known for her dedication to medicine and her approachable style of education and advocating for women's health.

In closing, I would like to share a story that I feel is why I wish I had this book 12 years ago when my own daughter started her periods. It was one of those days where everything seemed to be collapsing and I heard my daughter yell from the bathroom that she needed help. With her head poking out the door, she whispered 'I need a tampon'. I am an OBGYN, so I'm not sure why she whispered 'tampon', but I suppose having three younger brothers in the house was reason enough. As fate would have it, I was the only parent home and I ran to the car and drove to the local pharmacy to buy 'tampons' (I think I may have even whispered the word tampon in my head). I walked into the pharmacy confident as an OBGYN and down the aisle to discover a massive wall of tampons and pads. I was overwhelmed by the selection: brands, sizes, light days, heavy days, wings, applicator, no applicator – I began to sweat. I must have stood and stared at this looming wall of feminine products looking a bit lost, because an older woman walked up to me and put her hand on my arm: 'Do you need some help?' I looked over at her and said, 'Wow there is quite a selection, but I think I've got this.' She smiled and walked away knowing I had no idea what I was doing. When I got home and handed the box to my daughter I was greeted by a thankful face, and then as she closed the door I heard a scream, 'DAD!'

'What did you buy?' she said from behind the door.

'Ummmm' was all I could get out.

'Oh my god, these are huge, they won't fit,' she yelled.

In my nervous haste, staring at the wall of tampons, I chose a box that was for women with heavy periods, and as such they were larger and not made for a young girl.

The point of this story is that even as an OBGYN we often have a hard time relating to our own children and if I can make this mistake, I imagine others could as well. I wish I would have had this book, *Beautiful You*, before I went to the store, because I could have used Dr Kringoudis' advice. This book is not only a parenting treasure, it is a resource guide for young women needing the advice from someone they can trust. I know you will find this book as valuable as I have.

Shawn Tassone, MD PhD

Assistant Professor of Women's Health

University of Texas Dell Medical Center

America's Holistic Gynecologist

Austin TX

www.tassonemd.com

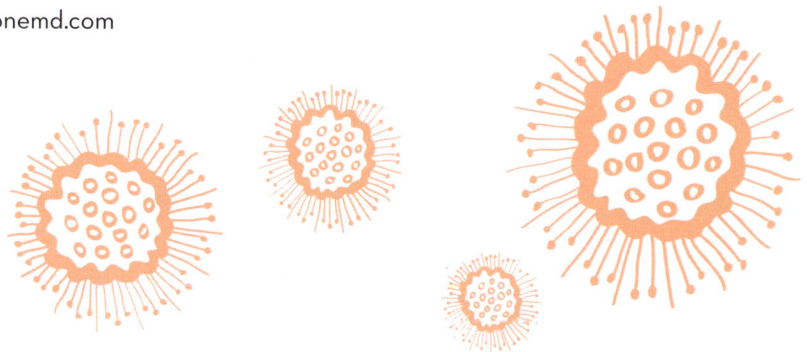

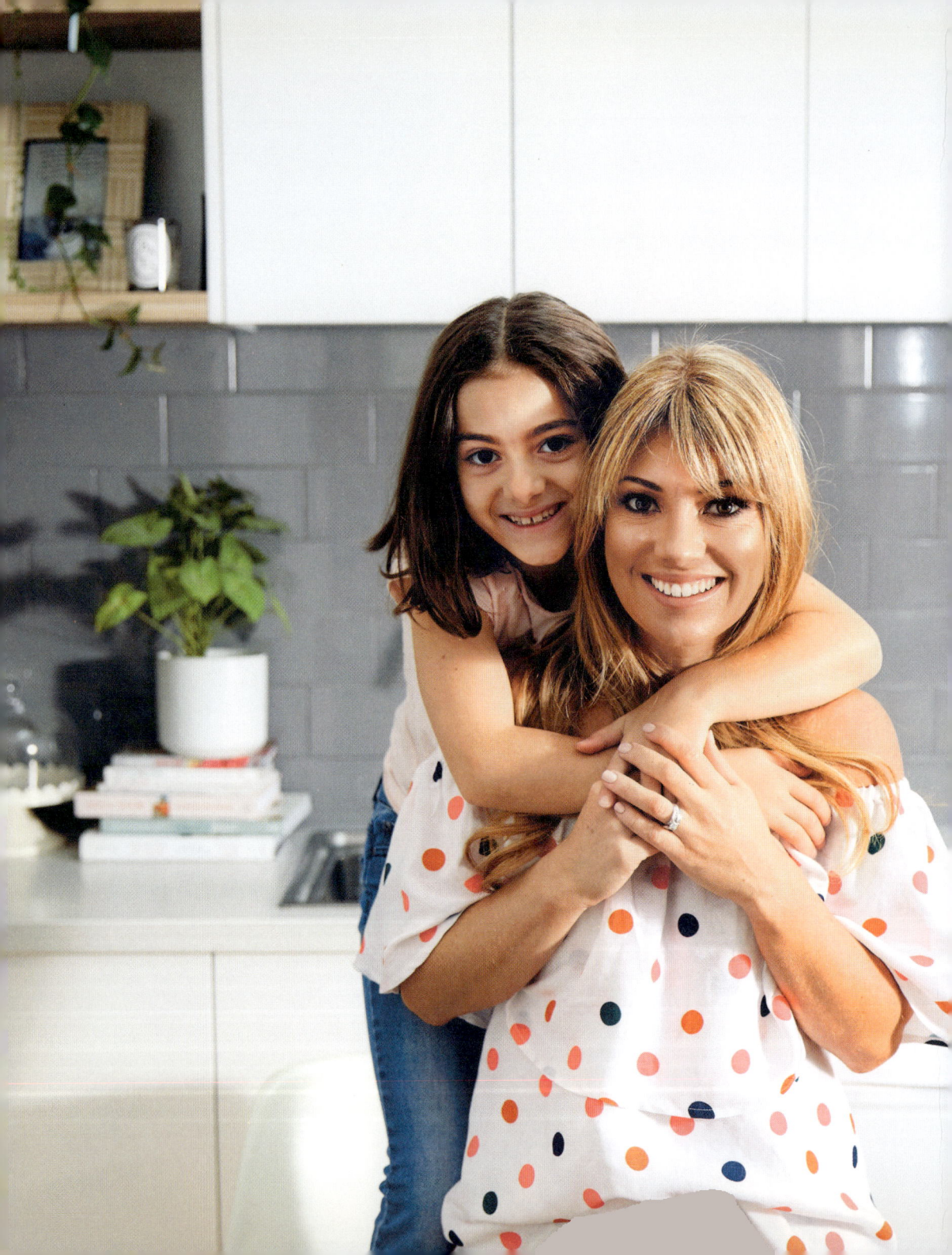

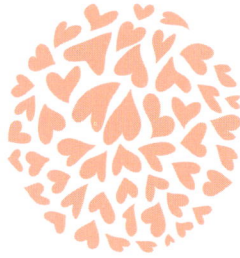

Introduction

In anticipation of my first period, I carried around a Stayfree pad in the bottom of my bag until the ends frayed. I wasn't really that keen for it to show up, but I sure didn't want it to come and I not be prepared, nor did I want to be the last of my friends to join the period club. I had visuals of a bloody mess 'down there' and couldn't even fathom the embarrassment that would come with it. I was also pretty nervous, mostly because I didn't want to be 'that girl' facing high school, needing to pretend to every other girl that I had tampons down pat. Finally, just a few weeks short of high school starting, it arrived. I remember walking out of the toilet, worried. I told Mum something bad had happened and I thought I needed to see a doctor. What I saw looked nothing like what I thought my period would actually look like. In fact, I didn't even associate what I saw with my period. And while this may be TMI (too much information) for an opening paragraph of this gorgeous book (if I may say so myself), my period looked nothing short of a murky, dirty mess in my undies.

In hindsight, I didn't really understand what it was all about – besides it being a sign that I was developing as a woman, or so my mum insisted. I didn't understand the importance of my period, no matter how many times I read the pamphlet Mum handed me when we had the 'birds and the bees' talk – and still to this day I don't understand what birds or bees have to do with my lady parts. I must have read those pages hundreds of times in fascination that my body was about to do all kinds of weird and wonderful things. I was actually obsessed with knowing more. Maybe I knew that someday, I would be talking about hormones every single day. I certainly didn't understand my menstrual cycle, I didn't know what hormones were – they sounded like an old lady who happened to moan way too much – and I wasn't prepared for the changes my body was about to go through either. Of course, it wasn't my mum's fault, she did a wonderful job with the resources she had found to at least try and show me what was happening on the inside (but more on that later).

PAIN AND DREAD

Eventually my period became something I started to dread. Pain began to creep in and learning to use a tampon was forced upon me when I woke up to my monthly surprise the very same morning we were having our end-of-year school breakup at the local swimming pools. I recall sitting in the bathroom trying to fit something the size of a small carrot into something that seemed the size of a pea. I couldn't figure it out and it seemed to burn like crazy and feel terribly uncomfortable. I really had no idea what I was doing. I asked myself many times, was it normal to feel like a child trapped inside this weird, almost lady's body?

It wasn't until many years later that I really started to learn about my menstrual cycle, about why acne started popping up everywhere or why my breasts grew at different speeds and hurt like crazy – as if I'd been repeatedly punched in the chest (why was the left one always smaller?). I never cared much about what it meant to be fertile or bothered to understand my body better, not only my period but the whole cycle. Truthfully, for years

I had no real idea. When I say years, I mean I'm still fascinated and I'm still learning about my body each and every day. It wasn't until I really started to observe the changes that my body would go through each month, and got super comfortable with myself, that I could actually stand back and watch in amazement, realising it had its own special groove.

I WANT TO HELP YOU UNDERSTAND YOU

What I want for you as a young woman is to really understand your body, your health and your hormones. I want to help you find your beauty both inside and out. I want to help take away the fear that you have towards your body and restore it with appreciation and overwhelming amazement for its special and intricate inner workings. I want to help you understand symptoms aren't payback or punishment for something you've done wrong in life, but are secret small warning signs telling you something needs attention. It's time for me to help you understand that if you don't look after your body, it won't love you back and this can show up in an array of symptoms and conditions, including endometriosis and Polycystic Ovarian Syndrome (PCOS) (more on that later), and pose a threat to your fertility someday. If we can understand that, most often, these health conditions are actually a direct result of how we are living our lives, we can quickly remedy the root cause of the problem rather than treating a by-product or symptoms. Finally, I want to share some awesome tips and tricks I wish somebody had told me, to help get you through these confusing years of early womanhood.

My absolute hope is that this book becomes your go-to, your place of discovery and a place you feel safe to open up the pages and really get to know yourself as a gorgeous human being. My hope is that this book begins to help you paint your own picture of you. Get comfortable with being different from the other women in your life. Though becoming a woman may be scary at first, you'll quickly learn there's a whole lot of fun ready to be had and that you deserve the best version of yourself, no matter what. Let's make it a beautiful journey, together.

I love that you are here and I love that we get to do this together. Let's get started, shall we?

In this book you will find a bunch of fun facts, frequently asked questions, and tips and tricks to have you all over your health and your happiness. After all, happiness is an inside job.

You are beautiful,
every day,
in every way.

Fill this page with things you love about yourself – list at least 5.

1.

2.

3.

4.

5.

6.

7.

8.

WORKSHEET: **HEALTH GOALS**

Let's get focused on where we are headed. I'd love for you to imagine the best version of you. What does she look like; how does she act or behave? Perhaps she's pain free or her eyes twinkle with health or she feels really comfortable in her own skin. **Whatever that may be for you, jot down several words that describe her.** We're going on a hunt to find her and bring her out into this big, beautiful world.

'You're in pretty good shape for the shape you are in.'

DR SEUSS

CHAPTER 1

Your hormones

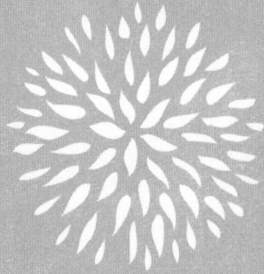

'Knowledge is such a gift.
By simply understanding
our body we immediately
take away any fear.'

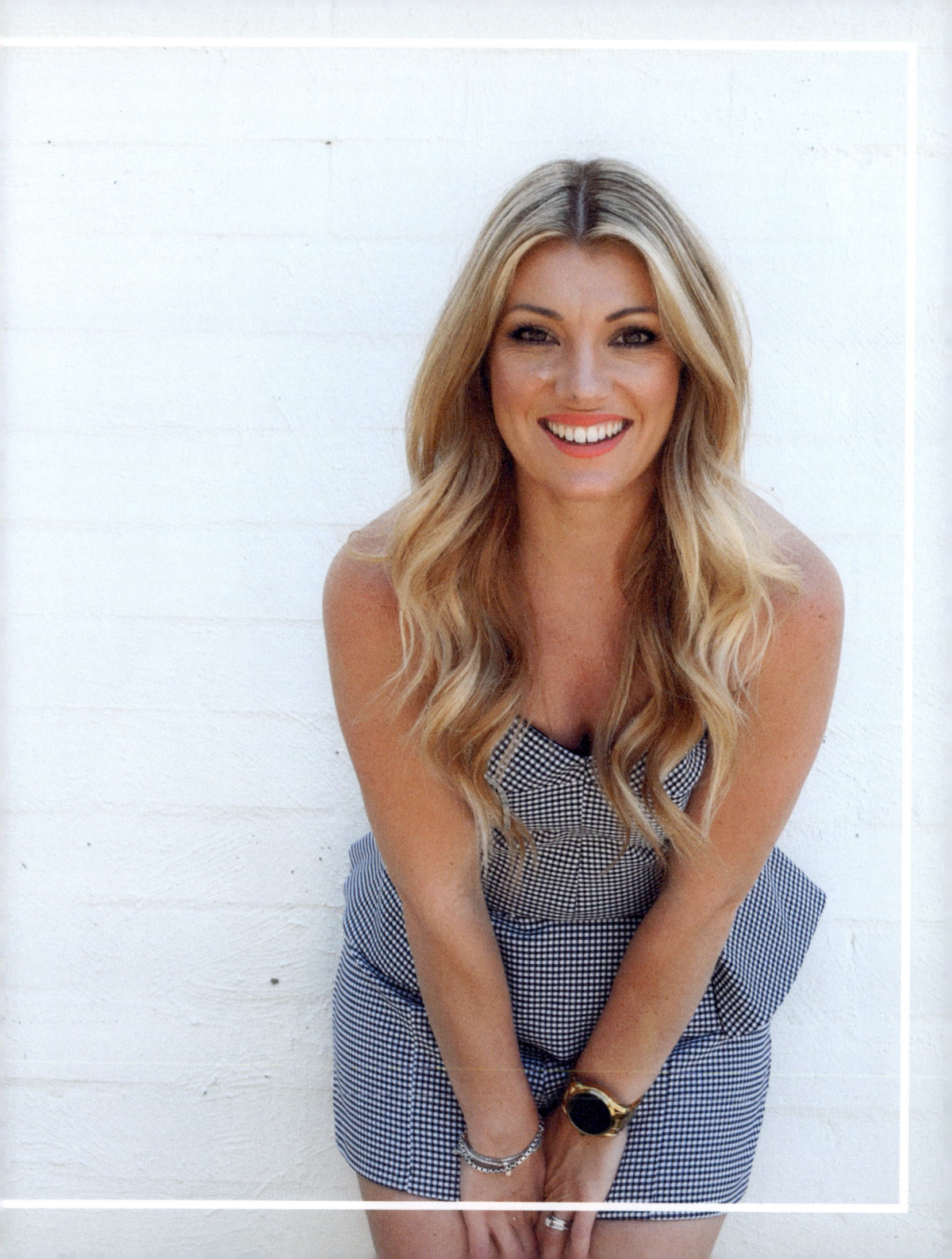

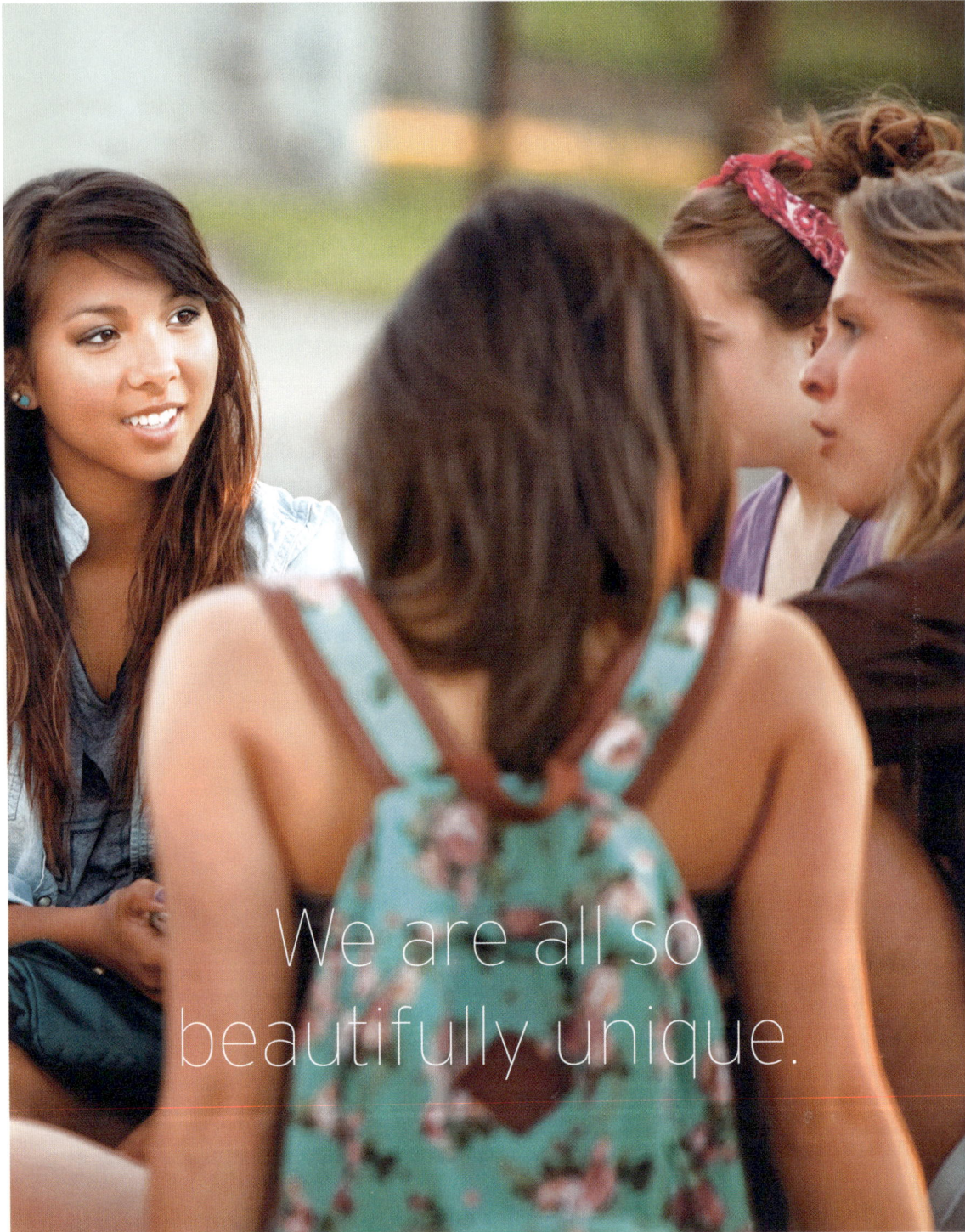

We are all so
beautifully unique.

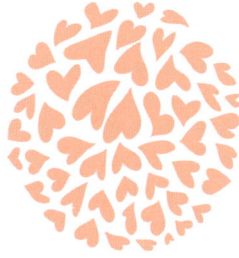

The real secret to a happier, healthier you!

YOU WILL LEARN:

• the role of major hormones (it's not as boring as it sounds, I promise)

• what your hormones are telling you (please tell me why I have acne!)

Can we agree on just one thing before we go on? You are totally amazing.
You have the world at your feet. You are beautiful – no matter what the
calendar says, we all are. Truth bomb: know it. In fact, you could even say it.
Right now, close your eyes and whisper to yourself, 'I am amazing.' Not once,
not twice, but three times over to really let it sink in. You are actually all that
and so much more. You have a whole big, wild life that's right there for you
to go and live. But it's scary at the same time – I know it, I've been there too.
When I think about everything I've ever been scared out of my pants about in
my life, I realise it's always been because of the fear of the unknown. It's our
natural sway – to worry about what we don't know, because it's nothing short

of frightening and I suppose worry is some kind of coping mechanism in an attempt to control a situation. But it doesn't really work. Worry just makes us tired and unwell, as you will learn.

But what if you could have special golden nuggets of useful and reassuring information that helped ease the load a little? To release the lid on the pressure, because once you understand something it's generally a-ok. The fear is gone and we know what's happening. That is my wish and it's totally possible.

Worry doesn't work; it just makes us tired and unwell.

Maybe you remember the first time you tackled algebra (seemed like if I didn't understand it, I was definitely from Mars). Perhaps you loved it and it all clicked or perhaps you were like me and had to work really hard at understanding it. It felt to me like if I didn't nail it, I was a failure. But thankfully I've learnt that nobody is a failure because we are all so beautifully unique and if you work out algebra isn't actually your thing, it's going to be ok. We don't all have to understand and fully embrace algebra because we aren't all going to be engineers. If we produced a world where we all turned up with the same occupation, each and every day, I don't know about you but I'd want out. How boring! But when it comes to your body – and we all have one of those – it's in our best interest to understand it, not necessarily on a physiological or cellular level but in a general sense of how we feel and act each day.

So let's understand a little about your hormones because they are like the master controller of YOU. If the word 'hormones' bores you, hear me out. I want you to know why you must begin to love your hormones: it's because

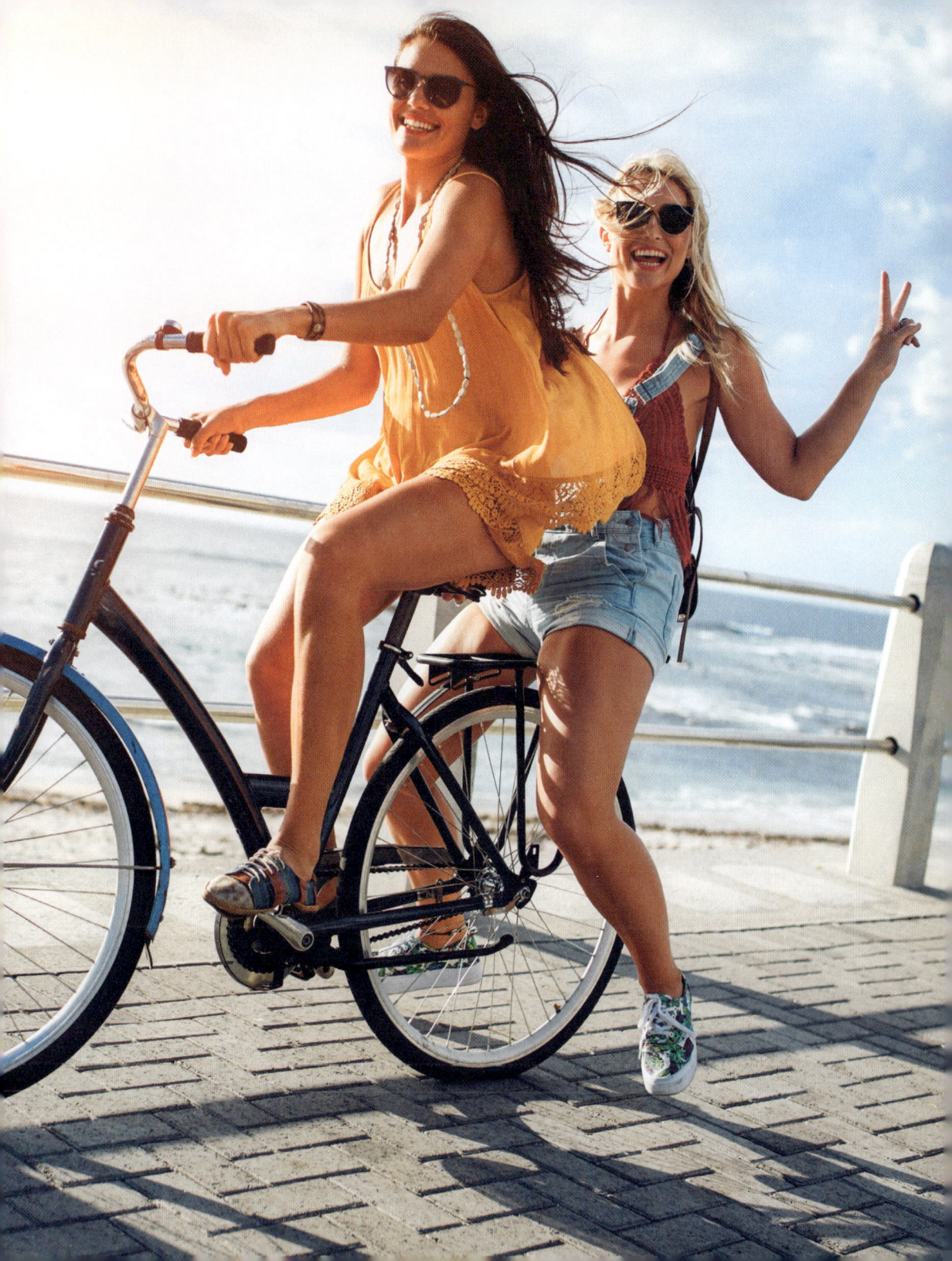

I want to keep it simple for you, so I've broken it right down. The most fascinating thing I see is how our hormones can influence physical changes. So next time you're feeling bloated, tired, pimply or puffy, your hormones might just have some answers for you!

Oestrogen

Your most feminine hormone mostly made in your ovaries, oestrogen is actually three hormones: oestradiol, oestrone and oestriol. Oestrogen controls your menstrual cycle (alongside progesterone mostly).

Oestradiol is the one we are most concerned with – it's responsible for our development as women (boobs, pubes and all), as well as our fertility. And while I know you're certainly not at an age of longing for babies yet, you'll want to keep that gift in check because applying the idea that it can be dealt with someday is fairly well outdated along with the iPhone 4 and snail mail. Truth is, you don't actually need to do much to preserve your fertility other than love your body and feed it right. We've adopted the idea that our bodies will generally be broken and we will need to fix them at some point in time but the magic lies in caring for yourself each and every day – and that's actually pretty simple, as you'll see. Anyway, back to oestradiol. It's also totally important for brain function, sleep and keeping our bones healthy. This is the hormone that is most related to any hormone imbalance problems like endometriosis (see Chapter 4).

Oestrone is produced in the ovaries as well as the fatty tissue of the body and in the adrenals too. Oestrone is one of the major hormones produced by menopausal women. Not something you're needing anytime soon but always good to have on your radar and also if Mum is reading this book! (Hi Mum.)

Oestriol is a type of oestrogen that is in full swing during pregnancy. In a non-pregnant woman, levels of oestriol are very low.

Progesterone

Also mostly produced in the ovaries, progesterone is the bomb! It's known as the calming hormone; it increases your metabolism (keeps your body weight in check) and also works as a brain hormone, boosting your 'feel good' hormones. Healthy progesterone can relieve symptoms like insomnia, and helps relieve stress or depression and move out excess fluid from the body. If you're low in progesterone, you can see symptoms like weight gain, anxiety, emotional issues, water retention and bloating, and long menstrual cycles.

Balanced oestrogen and progesterone really are the key to feeling happier and saying goodbye to a host of unwanted symptoms. Didn't I tell you your hormones unlock the key to feeling healthy, happy and awesome!

Testosterone

It's not just for boys! Without testosterone we can't make healthy hormones. Testosterone is also predominantly made in the ovaries of women. Excess testosterone can lead to weight gain, accelerated hair growth (which can be darker and thicker), acne and voice changes. Testosterone imbalance can be one of the main reasons we see Polycystic Ovarian Syndrome (PCOS).

These are our main sex hormones that contribute most to our menstrual cycles. There are a few more that are good to understand, especially when you are stacking up your symptoms to use as clues.

Cortisol

The stress hormone! It is released to help us cope with stress. If it remains 'turned on' over a period of time, it can really push our sex hormones out of balance and tends to win over progesterone, meaning it can cause terrible imbalance. As a result of this, it can be a contributor to raising oestrogen levels.

Adrenaline

Produced in the adrenal glands, adrenaline (also known as epinephrine) plays an important role in the fight or flight response. This means when you need to jump out of the way of a moving car, adrenaline kicks in, increasing blood flow to your muscles. Excess adrenaline can contribute to hormone imbalance due to ongoing stress. It's important to be able to keep stress in check for this reason.

Insulin

Produced in the pancreas, insulin responds to blood sugar to help you store energy. It assists the body in moving nutrients into the cells. Since high blood sugar can be problematic, insulin is a key player in maintaining health. Insulin resistance is often behind hormone imbalance like PCOS. It's an important player in hormone regulation. Over time your cells can become desensitised to insulin, which causes too much of it to sit outside of the cells rather than being utilised. This can force the ovaries to make too much testosterone, which contributes to imbalances like PCOS. Excess insulin is also behind type 2 diabetes.

DHEA

This is the queen of the hormones! DHEA stands for dehydroepiandrosterone. It's a steroid hormone produced in the adrenal glands. It can turn into many of our other sex hormones. It's also important to maintain youth, keeping our muscles strong; it gives us brainpower and helps with weight management and overcoming stress.

Melatonin

Made in the brain, melatonin is the sleep and body clock regulator. So if you find yourself tired and grumpy or your periods are all over the place, it may be because melatonin is being sacrificed. This hormone is produced in darkness, which is why it's so important to sleep when it's night-time and in the dark too!

Serotonin

This neurotransmitter is said to be responsible for happiness and general wellbeing. (We all need this to be in balance!) Produced predominantly in the gastrointestinal tract, it's important for hormone balance and all-round wellness.

Thyroid hormones

Every single cell in your body requires your thyroid to work properly, meaning if it is out of kilter even in the slightest, the symptoms are wide and varied. Your thyroid is very sensitive to stress. Think of your thyroid like your internal thermostat. It regulates your metabolism and plays a vital role in keeping you feeling perky and vibrant.

Melanocyte-Stimulating Hormone

A big name given to a group of hormones, known collectively as MSH, this group is produced in response to UV sunlight (or radiation). MSH helps produce pigmentation, giving us our skin colour, hair colour and eye colour.

Growth hormone

This is the growth stimulator that is released in the early stages of our sleep, which is why it is so important to get adequate rest, especially as young adults. It also helps with repair of our body, as well as brain function and metabolism.

Adiponectin

Secreted from your fat cells, adiponectin is a protein hormone that helps regulate insulin and reduce inflammation. This is important for those with PCOS, where there is not enough adiponectin being secreted. Insulin resistance is something we will tuck into later, but excess insulin will lead to a host of issues including weight gain, and can often be at the core of PCOS too.

HORMONES

HORMONES AFFECT YOUR BOWELS

HORMONES AFFECT ENERGY

HORMONES AFFECT YOUR WEIGHT

HORMONES AFFECT BODY FAT

HORMONES AFFECT YOUR SKIN

HORMONES AFFECT YOUR MOODS

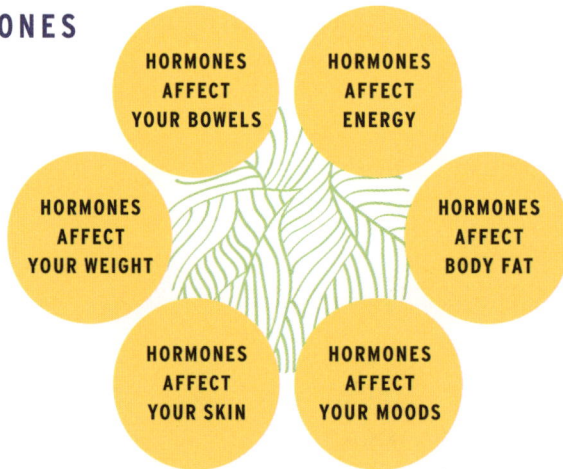

Remember, your symptoms are your clues. It's good to understand exactly what your hormones can be telling you at various times. Hormones may be affecting your energy levels, body fat, skin, moods, and even your bowels. When we can understand that each sign is a result of our body not working properly, we can act on the core issue to effect change.

When our hormones are balanced, our body works well, the organs function properly and we feel good! But when that isn't in tip-top shape it can have massive effects all over, and you may especially feel this in your energy levels and moods.

HOW HORMONES CAN AFFECT WEIGHT LOSS

WHEN WE EAT FOOD OUR HORMONAL RESPONSE DETERMINES WHETHER WE STORE FAT OR BURN FAT

WEIGHT AND FAT LOSS IS REGULATED BY HORMONES

THERE ARE MANY INVOLVED, BUT THE MAIN ONES ARE INSULIN, GLUCAGON, CORTISOL AND THYROID HORMONES

HOW HORMONES CAN AFFECT YOUR SKIN

PSORIASIS

ECZEMA

NOSE BLEEDS

RED SKIN AND SWELLING

FACIAL HAIR

ACNE

SYMPTOMS OF HORMONE IMBALANCE

- Acne or rashes

- Amenorrhea (missing period after 15 or 16 years of age)

- Anxiety

- Back acne

- Bloating/gas

- Depression

- Dysmenorrhea (painful periods)

- Excessive cravings

- Excessive hair growth (on breasts or stomach)

- Hair loss

- Headaches

- Heavy bleeding

- Insomnia

- Irregular menstrual cycles

- Long menstrual cycles

- Nosebleeds

- Pelvic pain

- Premenstrual Tension (PMT)

- Recurrent infections or illness

- Sluggish bowels

- Spotting

- Velvety skin patches in creases

- Weight gain

WHY HAVE A PERIOD AT ALL?

I get it; it's inconvenient, it feels like it comes around all the time and it often brings with it an overloaded Mack Truck full of symptoms ranging from acne and pain to loose bowels and irritability. But I'm encouraging you to learn that menstruation is absolute evidence of health – if it comes with a trailer load of problems, this is your body's very own unique way of begging you for mercy and to darn well do something about it.

When your body is in good balance, you'll find fewer niggly symptoms; you may find your cycles are more regular and not too painful or troublesome. But when symptoms of irregular, heavy, light, long or absent periods set in alongside headaches, acne or premenstrual tension (PMT) or pain, your body is literally screaming out really loudly for help.

Your period provides a window into the internal environment of your body.

Too Much Information? As TMI as it sounds, I want you to have as much info at your fingertips as possible – I'm asking for permission to get really detailed, which may leave you a little grossed out, but this information is essential for you, in this lifetime at least.

Your period menses (aka blood) is chock-full of immune cells and is, interestingly, the only blood in your body that doesn't clot. A scientist by the name of Margie Profet concluded that there's more to your period than just an 'inconvenient' bleed every 28 days or so. It isn't a design fault; in fact it's a perfect situation (it always is). When your period flows, it cleanses the uterus, cervix and vagina with this clean, antiviral, antibacterial blood, thus providing you with an inbuilt sanitising system. Blocking this natural flow may be a disaster for more reasons than we once thought. It makes sense each month to shed the uterine lining to cleanse and then get ready to repeat the process. For many women this isn't necessarily the case, be it that they don't get a regular period or they are using hormonal birth control to stop the period. The trick with all things in life (your body is no different) is to work with it, not against it. Wishing your period away may not be as wonderful as you think AND if you are wishing it away because it's horrible, let's sort that out, shall we?

Your 'normal' period

There are so many variations to what a 'normal' cycle should look like, but for the purpose of clarity, I'm going to talk about how it should look in a 'perfect case' scenario. We can discuss variations a little later on. Your period can provide you with so much information about your body.

This is how a typical month should roll around. I want to explain the ovulation chart (see page 39) thoroughly, so I'm going to break it down to simple town. Remember, this is all a 'rough' guide in terms of time frames. All women will vary – and that is perfectly normal.

Ok, so it is fairly standard that the period will last anywhere from 2 to 7 days. In the clinic, I like to see a period be no longer than 5 days. Bleeding for too long can certainly leave the body depleted or be a possible sign of too much oestrogen (since oestrogen helps build the lining, it makes sense that more of it makes the lining thicker and therefore more needs to be shed) and therefore it is important that blood loss isn't too significant. It should be no more than 6 tablespoons in total – not that you need to measure it but for some women using menstrual cups, you may be able to gauge just how much blood is lost each and every month! In any case, it's a great guide (however, it's difficult to tell with the standard of sanitary products nowadays).

Work
with it, not
against it.

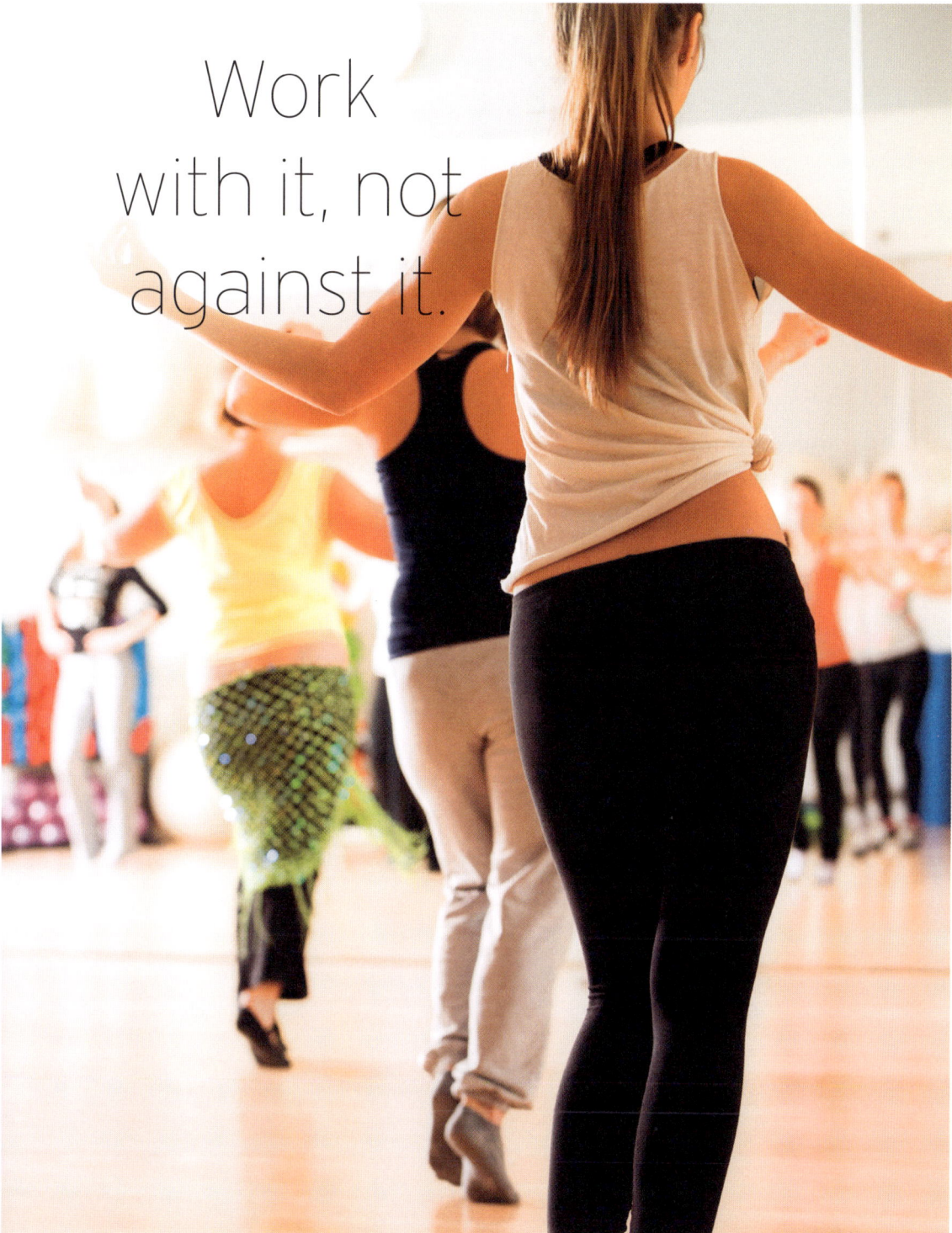

Should you experience a 1-day bleed that is dry and dark without proper flow, there is a chance you aren't actually ovulating but experiencing a hormone bleed. It's a good idea to speak to your healthcare professional and have a blood test done to see what might be going on. Start by confirming ovulation.

Dr Shawn Tassone, an OBGYN with a focus on integrative medicine, describes this anovulatory bleeding really well, likening oestrogen to water and plant food (fertiliser) and progesterone to the lawn mower. If you are constantly watering the grass, it will continue to grow to the point where it outgrows its supply and begins to keel over. This is what happens when you don't have the lawn mower (progesterone) but you experience a bleed; it is actually a result of the overgrowth and build up resulting in shedding, but not a true period. These bleeds are often characteristically lighter and have less of a flow.

Now, from this point on is where the fun starts. To put this into practice, you will need to learn to feel what your body is telling you (and begin to use the diary at the back of this book). As grey and 'woo woo' as it sounds, you can actually 'feel' ovulation via your cervical fluid patterns. Here's how. Perhaps you've worked out that you know the moment when your period comes because you've recognised that it feels a certain way 'down there' (typically it feels wet and warm around the opening of the vagina). Ovulation is mostly the same, although rather than it feeling wet and warm, it feels wet and cold. I'm not talking about how it feels between your fingertips either. I'm referring to the sensation you feel around the opening of the vagina. It becomes more about not necessarily what you can physically see in terms of cervical mucus, but more about what you can actually sense.

Typically, one should have several 'dry' days (that is, without any cervical fluid or mucus) before starting to notice a small amount (days 6–9), followed by the feeling of moistness (days 10–12). See the ovulation chart on the following page. This can last for several days until you begin to feel signs of optimal fertility – clear and stretchy cervical mucus – remember it feels wet and cold. Cervical mucus is essential for conception. It is the sperm's mode of transport up to the eagerly waiting egg. The cervix secretes this vital fertile mucus. When the semen is ejaculated into the vagina, the sperm will make its way up to the cervical crypts (where the mucus is secreted from) where it stays for a bit, and takes a little rest to be fed and rejuvenated (I find it hilarious that it is already hungry!), before it continues on up to meet the egg. If you take a look at fertile cervical mucus under a microscope, it appears as many little channels – unlike infertile mucus which is a hash tag-like pattern, making it impossible for the sperm to swim through. This is why fertile mucus is essential for conception. Fertile mucus can last for several days while the body gears up to ovulate. **Ovulation isn't the day you see the most cervical fluid – it is the LAST day that you see or feel it.**

So here in the ovulation chart, you see it is cycle day 15 that ovulation occurs, even though there has been wet and cold cervical fluid present for 3 days. It is the final day that this wet feeling is experienced that marks ovulation. The tricky part is that it isn't something you will know until after the event, which makes it totally frustrating. However, as you begin to observe your body's signs and symptoms, you'll become more able to know what's going on and be able to follow your patterns, helping to determine your ovulation window.

For women with happy and healthy ovaries, there is generally a line or 'string like' formation of follicles that sit happily in succession on each of the ovaries – like cabs in a rank, each is a little 'riper' than the one that follows, gearing up for ovulation. Ovulation is when the most mature, ripened follicle is triggered to be released by a surge in Lutenising Hormone (LH). It is at the time of its release that your body is most fertile as the follicle or 'egg' begins to make its way from the ovary, down the fallopian tube, ready for fertilisation – the act of sperm meeting the egg as a result of sexual intercourse.

Fertilisation generally happens within a fallopian tube and eventually continues to make its way to the endometrium (uterine lining), where it implants around 5 days after ovulation. This is the early stage of pregnancy. Failing the event of fertilisation, the body will get ready for the endometrial lining to shed and repeat the process all over again: this is marked each month by your period.

Ovulation can be sometimes early and sometimes late, especially as your hormones find their groove. When it is repeatedly early (less than 21 days), repeatedly late (over 35 days) or irregular, it may be an indication that your hormones are begging for a little TLC. The trick is to understand your cycles to decode exactly what is going on. Your cycle tells you so much about the internal landscape of your sex hormones.

Now, from cycle day 16 right through to 28 is when the hormone progesterone is in full swing and you may notice there is very little or no mucus. This is normal. During this time (it is called the luteal phase), your body is busy either implanting that embryo or preparing for your period. However, you may notice a little mucus or discharge nearing the end of this phase, which is completely normal and the result of a second surge of progesterone. Should you sense mucus throughout the luteal phase, that's ok too. You may notice that it's typically drier and certainly doesn't come with the same sensation felt during ovulation. It may be more a case of what you see when you wipe after going to the bathroom or as residue in your underwear, not so much the wet and cold sensation mentioned earlier.

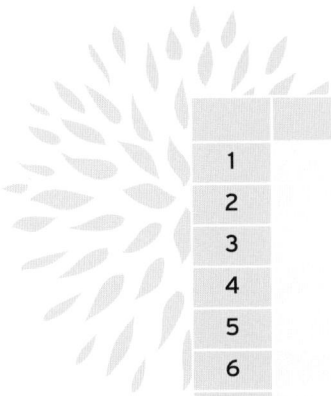

DAYS		INFORMATION
1	Period - heavy	Pain
2	Period - medium	
3	Period - medium	
4	Period - light	
5	Spotting	
6	Dry	
7	Dry	
8	Dry	
9	Dry	
10	Moist	
11	Moist	
12	Moist	
13	Wet	
14	Wet	
15	Wet	Ovulation
16	Dry	
17	Dry	
18	Dry	
19	Dry	
20	Dry	
21	Dry	
22	Dry	
23	Dry	
24	Dry	
25	Dry	Tender breasts
26	Dry	PMS
27	Dry	PMS
28	Dry	PMS and irritability

*This is a sample chart. Your cycle might be different.

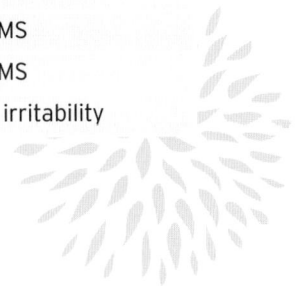

Discharge is very normal and is generally a sign of a healthy vagina. How much you have and the particular smell can vary.

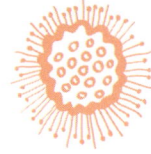

Discharge that is white or clear without odour is a sign of healthy vaginal flora. Discharge that is coloured (yellow or green) or has a rotten or fishy smell may be a sign of a deeper issue.

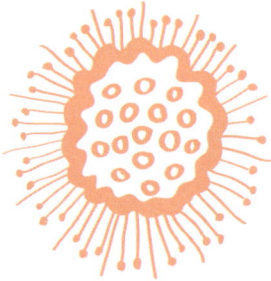

How you smell 'down there' absolutely varies from woman to woman. This is reflective of your own unique bacteria, diet, lifestyle, the material you expose your intimate parts to, how often you wash as well as your body secretions and your own personal smell (we all have this – it's a good thing!). Using organic cotton or non-synthetic materials can be a good idea to help keep your vaginal flora healthy. It's very normal for you to have your own unique odour and is nothing to be worried about, unless it has an offensive smell. Your vagina also secretes pheromones, which are chemicals that are said to initiate excitement and sexual interest, innately helping us attract a suitable partner. All animals secrete pheromones for the same reason – just another way our bodies are so clever!

Handy info for years to come...

Should your cycles be a bit out of sorts well into your 20s – say ovulation is occurring earlier or later – it's something that is good to investigate a little further. As with everything in life, however, there is always a reason. It may mean that you're experiencing hormone imbalance and the consequence down the track may be 'sub-fertility'. This doesn't mean you are infertile, it means that you have the potential to be fertile, but hormonally you are imbalanced and in this very moment, your body may not support a healthy pregnancy. So for example, ovulating on cycle day 9 may be a problem, since it means an immature follicle is being released – making it almost impossible to be fertilised. Or maybe as another example, your luteal phase (from ovulation to the period time) is too short, meaning that if there is a growing embryo, it can't continue to grow because it isn't being supplied hormonally with all it requires. In almost all cases, we can treat this and begin to improve fertility. I have a swag of tricks that can be applied in these circumstances. See pages 44-49.

Over the first few years of menstruation, your cycles may be a little scratchy and this is generally nothing to worry about, in fact it's pretty normal. What isn't ok, however, is if they come with a kit full of symptoms; you will certainly want to explore their deeper meaning. And while period pain may be something we've been told is normal, it certainly doesn't need to be there and is an issue of modern living. See Chapter 4 for more on painful periods.

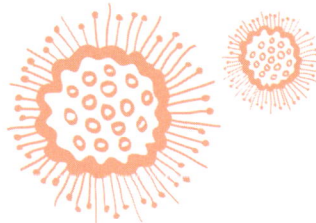

As women,
we have many
superpowers.

Your hormones according to the seasons

As women, we have many superpowers. I think one of the greatest barriers I observe in my clinic is the pressure that comes with being a woman in a patriarchal world. We can be persuaded to act in a predominantly masculine manner, because men may 'appear' to get the job done (even though we actually do an excellent job too) and we may try to match their style. It's when we begin to operate out of this place that we lose sight of what is innately us. Men have a role just as women do. Do we really want to be men? No. But if we actually tapped in to our own essence, and felt the equally solid voice, I believe we would be in a different place. I believe women need to take their power through their femaleness by embracing it rather than denying it.

Women can behave like men and this is where I think there is an issue, because it's not being true to ourselves. As women, we are nurturers by nature – not only may we care for our own children if and when that time arrives, but equally our natural state is to care for all those around us, extending to other family members as well as friends, co-workers and other loved ones. The real gem would be if we worked out how to use our hormones to our advantage; I wonder if we'd have every XY chromosome on the planet buckling in and listening up. It's just a thought ...

Which brings me to this: **Understanding your hormones as a woman may be your very own unique superpower.**

UNDERSTANDING THE CYCLES ACCORDING TO THE SEASONS

The first place to start with this is to understand the cycles according to the seasons. You might be surprised to learn that men have cycles too – driven by testosterone, they cycle each and every day. The bonus for them is that these cycles tend to weave in with a typical work day. Women, however, very obviously cycle too, not only through the day, but most importantly throughout a month (or thereabouts). That's a lot of difference right there and we've only touched the tip of the iceberg.

This 'secret squirrel business' of our cycles as our superpower is very useful, and the circadian rhythm (our day and night 24-hour clock in which we are all cycling around) as well as our menstrual rhythm are both important to our health. Also important is how your brain (via the hypothalamus, which lies just above the pituitary gland at the base of your brain) and your adrenals (which are found on top of the kidneys and secrete your main stress hormones) all communicate – this is known as the hypothalamic-pituitary-adrenal axis or HPA axis.

Our cycles are our superpower.

I liken our cycles to a window into our reproductive hormones. How our cycles play out each month can tell us a lot about what is going on internally. Say we experience pain in the middle of the cycle or we frequently see our periods arrive a few days early. These little clues are like feedback from our body that our hormones may need some extra care. I like to divide up the cycle into phases or better still, seasons. Your menstrual cycle according to the seasons (and to use to your advantage) looks like this:

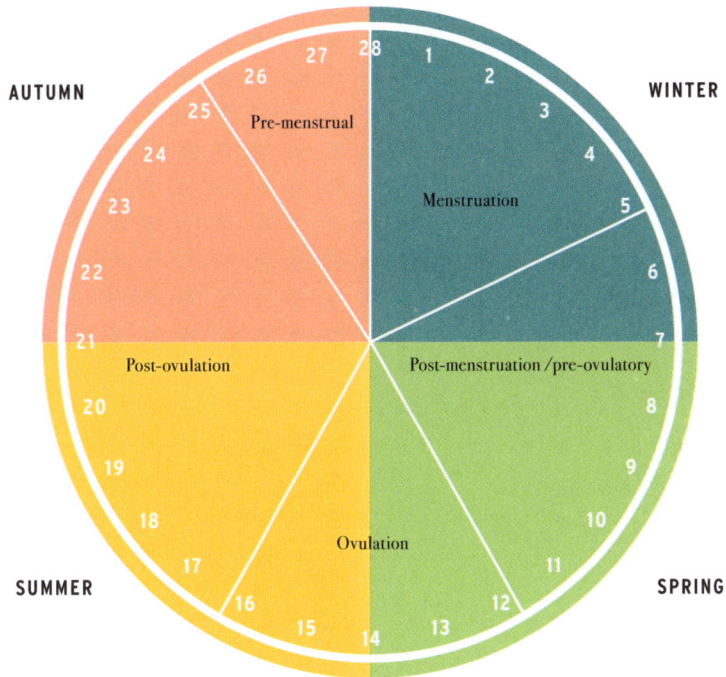

AUTUMN

WINTER

Pre-menstrual

Menstruation

Post-ovulation

Post-menstruation/pre-ovulatory

SUMMER

SPRING

Ovulation

1 2 3 4 5 6 7 8 9 10 11 12 13 14 15 16 17 18 19 20 21 22 23 24 25 26 27 28

WINTER

The menstrual stage facts

- This phase may last 3 days or it may last 7 (any longer and we need to talk).
- In this phase our hormones are at their lowest as the period starts.
- Oestrogen begins to rise as this phase goes by.
- Appetite may be low at this time (not like the week prior).
- Including warm and nourishing foods at this time is useful, as well as some dark chocolate for blood building – so Traditional Chinese Medicine (TCM) but I love it.
- During this phase it is important to go gently with movement and lifestyle.

- Spiritually, you may notice you are more centred and connected, and things feel 'deeper'; even your emotions may be like this, too.
- It's the time to stop and just be, trying not to push on just because the world tells you to.
- Spend more time on your own, be less social and even say no to things.
- Rest when needed, 'nap on tap'.

SPRING

The post-menstrual/pre-ovulation stage facts

- Oestrogen is building, progesterone is low but begins to rise and testosterone is rising in preparation for ovulation.
- During this time it is best to consume wholefoods, especially plant foods to nourish the body after the hibernation of the winter phase.
- Your energy is increasing and you feel light and bright.
- This is the time to get social, take holidays and attend or arrange important events. This fresh energy makes you more adventurous, too.
- It's your ultimate time to network.
- It's the time in your work to act and get new projects started.
- Clear away the clutter, fix the house or your room, and create space for the freshness arriving. Setting yourself up now makes the difference for the rest of the cycle.

SUMMER

The ovulation stage facts

- The hormones are high as oestrogen and testosterone peak before the soar of progesterone.
- Your digestion generally feels amazing at this point. You may also crave salty foods.

- Exercise at this time of the cycle feels awesome; you may find you feel stronger and more resilient than any other time in your cycle.
- You may find you need to really nurture the important relationships during this phase.
- Your libido (sexual desire) peaks and there is a heightened external sexual energy. Makes total sense, since innately you're ovulating for the purpose of procreation!
- This time of the cycle is also where you want to connect with your loved ones for some time together - pick up the phone to chat or support them in some way.

AUTUMN

The premenstrual stage facts

- Oestrogen (and progesterone eventually) levels dive if there isn't a fertilised egg.
- Your appetite moves in - carbs and sugar seem to be on the top of the list.
- It is a time in the cycle where it is more important to be aware of alcohol and sugar intake - both can cause chaos with your period due to the inflammation they bring.
- Exercise is important during autumn as it can assist with any premenstrual symptoms. Sex also can be useful to increase uterine blood flow and manage any pain, but of course you're not going to nab the nearest guy just to ease your period pain; more on this in later chapters.
- You may find yourself needing to go gently and you begin to turn inwards.
- Some find that the 'inner mean girl' shows up in this window. Do your best to let go of any negative ego that's rearing its head.
- Great practices to incorporate in autumn are warm baths, movies and

massages. Women are no longer fertile in the autumn stage, so I encourage you to partake in gentle exercise to alleviate any PMS symptoms.

• At home, clean up, create space and focus on letting go, all in preparation for your winter phase.

So how do you play big if you're waiting for your period? It's all about how we use this to our advantage. Some may say planning in and around your menstrual cycle is a good idea to help you get the most out of using your hormones to your advantage – for example if you have a presentation or a big event, try timing it for the summer phase when you are ovulating and the most 'out there'. This is wonderful in theory and an absolute bonus if luck has it fall at this time, although not always possible. Newsflash: sadly, the rest of the world doesn't actually revolve around your menstrual cycle. If only! If your periods are terrible, then it's time to sort them out but it is also important to read the signs and look at why you aren't feeling great throughout the cycles. I am, of course, always going to say let's fix your period!

You can use your hormones to your advantage.

So what are the benefits of having a menstrual cycle? The natural physical shifts that happen may be your secret weapon for life! Here are some examples.

Late follicular phase

This is when oestrogen and testosterone are high. There is reasonably good data to show you are going to be most productive, and this is the time to be your most 'masculine' self. Highest libido is also generally experienced here (or at least should be). This is also when you have the most energy.

Luteal phase

This is when there is high progesterone and relatively high oestrogen levels. In this time you may find yourself more intuitively aware and focused, and may find it easier to connect with other women. Thinking about how to use this to sway things your way may be very useful!

Building in times and giving ourselves permission for appropriate rest may also work to your advantage, but equally it's what you do in your down time. You see, rest and recovery is just as important as ticking boxes and making gains. It's about the ebbs and flows, and when you skip phases you most certainly can't continue at your best.

We need to allow for the ebbs and flows. It's unmaintainable if we don't; we end up getting fatigued, cranky and burnt out and our productivity plummets, reaching an all-time low. You may feel this as extreme fatigue or find that your period literally puts you on your butt for a few days. But also, we have these same ebbs and flows built in to our own natural feminine rhythm – these natural ups and downs – and when we don't have this awareness, we might try to fight against it, which leaves us feeling completely exhausted and unproductive. This may be the secret to enhancing our ability to function as women, and is certainly something men do not have. Using it to our advantage is a total game-changer. **If we are paying attention, there are benefits that can come from being aware of where you are in the cycle.**

Now this is all happy days until you need to show up on a day that your cycle wants you to rest (like the first day of your period). But if you are aware that this might happen and you are well versed in your job or the task you need to perform, you can build around the experience to make sure you nail it.

Start by doing as little as possible on 'game day' but focus on that very one thing you need to be achieving.

And here are a few tools to get you there:

- Get more sleep the night before and if possible, sleep in that day.
- Add in appropriate supplements, such as good quality magnesium, fish oil capsules (if you can take the oil, I salute you) and something like echinacea, which is known for its ability to sharpen the brain and improve cognitive thinking. It may be useful to check with your healthcare professional before taking supplements to ensure they are right for you. Not all supplements are made the same and quality matters. You can easily work out quality by the price – you get what you pay for (and nobody likes funky fish oil anyway).
- Practise good self care: take a nice shower, eat super good food and just take good care of you.

If you can set everything up to prepare yourself as if it is still a rest and recovery day, then this can soon become a little hack. After all, if it was up to nature, technically you're working on a rest day. This can be used for everything – when you have high-pressure tasks, plan around them and effectively build this into your cycle.

The other trick is being tuned in to your body and charting and watching what is going on and how you feel each month and each cycle. Who knows, you might feel best when you are actually bleeding or in the pre-period window. Be sure to start to use the diary in the back of this book! It's going to help you to understand your body on an entirely new level.

TESTING TESTING ... 123

You might wonder when the best time to head off for testing might be. Your doctor will best guide you but a Cervical Screening Test (the replacement test for pap smears) is generally recommended from the age of 25 and then every two years thereafter. However, if you have unusual bleeding, discharge or pain, please seek advice. Testing any time outside of the period is what I would recommend for such screening.

Sex hormone tests – say to see if you are ovulating or have enough sex hormones – are typically performed on the 21st day of your cycle. This is because if you have regular menstrual cycles, you should have ovulated by this time – if your tests tell you that you haven't, it's time to dig deeper. Your hormones also take time to find their groove and testing prematurely may cause unnecessary concern. If your menstrual cycles haven't settled by the time you are 18, then it may be a good time to test, otherwise know that it is very normal to have irregular cycles in your teen years.

CHAPTER 2

Your mindset

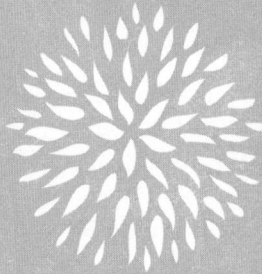

'Once your mindset changes,
everything on the outside
will change along with it.'

STEVE MARABOLI

Life, the Truth, and Being Free

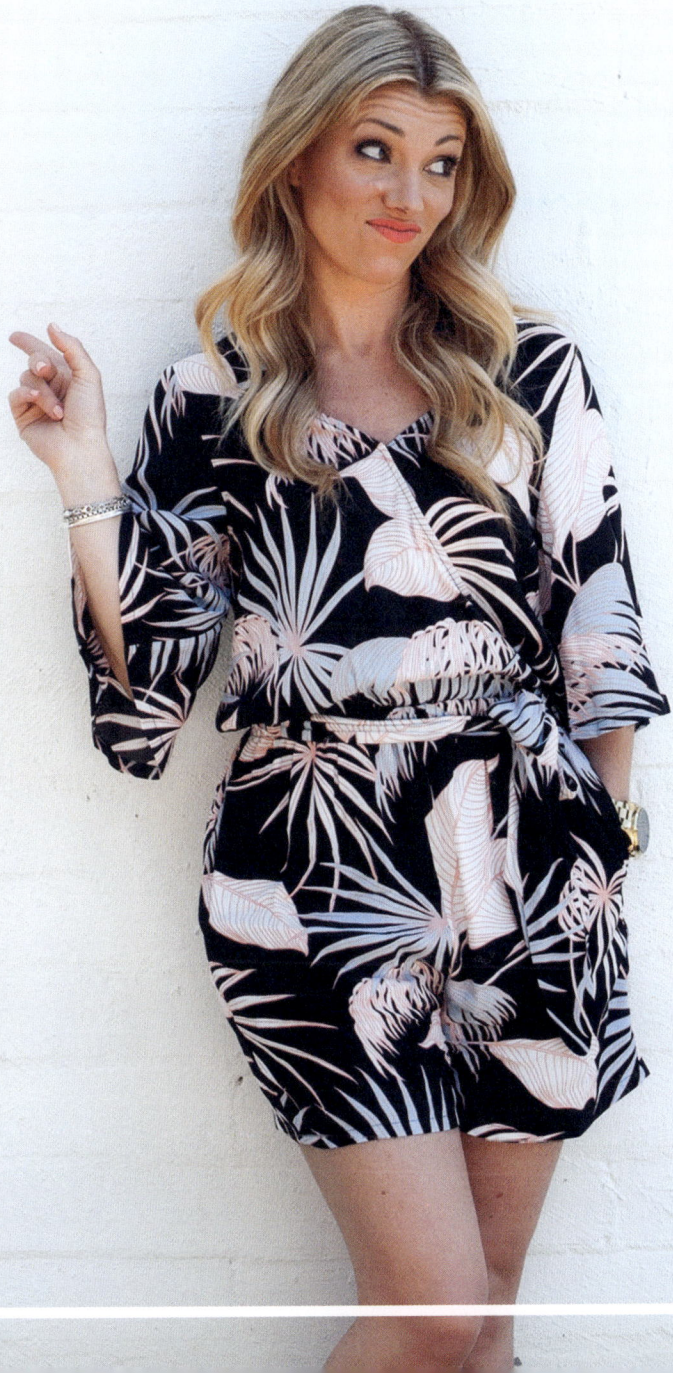

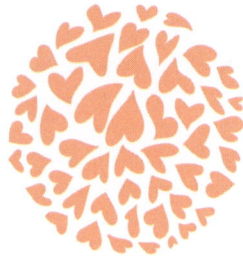

Switching it on to grow and glow

YOU WILL LEARN:

• how to get what you want

• that using your intuition becomes your superpower

There are three kinds of stress: internal stress (inside your body), external stress (environmental and lifestyle that exist outside of you) and mental stress (your mind). The key is understanding all three for better health and wellbeing.

Have you ever dressed up for a party or event and you felt like you had it all going on? The world's on your side, you feel good, you look amazing, everything is working for you. Girlfriend – you've got it all going on! Put yourself in the same dress, same hair, same makeup, but at another date – and you can experience the polar opposite. But why? You're wearing the same gorgeous dress, same heels, same makeup; but you look in the mirror and wonder where you went wrong. You feel perhaps bloated or frumpy, even your legs don't look the same when you're facing the mirror (trust me, they're still beautiful). There are several factors to consider in these circumstances but one of the most important is your mindset and attitude. You see, your mindset can either take you to exactly where you want to go or in the absolute opposite direction, no matter how bloated or frumpy you may feel.

What we focus on, expands. When you focus on the goodness in your life, you make more of it.

The saying 'what we focus on, expands' rings true. One of my first business mentors shared this quote with me and it resonated so deeply (I can only assume she heard it from Oprah Winfrey first!). That first time you wore the outfit, you were so excited, there was perhaps build up and you had that glow about yourself that can only come from having your eye on the goal. Who knows, maybe you were bloated, but it did not matter one bit, because you felt really good. Second time round, the excitement just wasn't there and quite possibly this time, rather than focusing on all the goodness that was, you could only see the opposite.

We can actually apply this to everything in life. Our mindset is one of our greatest tools when we learn to nurture it, to take us exactly where we want to go. The trick is knowing how, which may sound easier said than done. But if nurtured well, this can rapidly become your slipstream to ease all areas of your life. Of course, it is completely healthy and normal to experience an array of emotions – we can't be 100% happy all of the time. That's not reality, nor is it actually healthy. Experiencing the highs and not-so-highs of life is all part of growing; you might be frustrated to learn that it actually never ends – but it is what we do when we recognise we aren't feeling so great that counts most.

We get better at it the more we practise. **Emotions can manifest as physical symptoms anywhere in your body but very commonly they affect your reproductive system. Period pain is a perfect example of this.**

We may fall into the trap of becoming perpetually numb, because our clever (or not-so-clever) minds somehow worked out it might seem easier not to feel deeply and to shut down, rather than to sink our teeth into emotions that can be painful and heartbreaking. Feeling into each corner of emotions as they bubble also quickly becomes another trick in managing health better, even though it may not seem that way ... yet. Many experts argue that when emotions aren't experienced fully they can physically manifest in other more substantial ways, such as in illness or disease.

This manifests in the fact that all emotions, no matter how messy, must not only be felt and dealt with, but be seen as a gift towards gaining better health. Traditional Chinese Medicine (TCM) also dives further into this idea that if there is a recurrent emotion that is constantly tugging at your heartstrings, it may be a sign of internal disharmony or imbalance. It may be this same recurrent emotion we try and shoo away (but keeps on knocking on your chest) that is actually providing clues into which organ may be next in line for some tender loving care. Chinese Medicine theory categorises these as follows:

RECURRENT EMOTIONS AND ASSOCIATED ORGANS

ORGAN	EMOTION	SYMPTOMS
Liver	Anger, jealousy, envy, frustration	• Impaired digestion due to bile production imbalance • Decreased liver detoxification
Spleen (aka gut)	Worry, anxiety, hatred	• Irregular or loose bowels • Digestive upset
Lung	Sadness, depression	• Recurrent respiratory issues or poor immunity • Persistent low-grade cough • Constipation • Unresolved grief
Kidney	Fear, stress, depression	• Nervous system becomes stressed • Low libido • Increased acidity • General fatigue
Heart	Overjoy, impatience	• Palpitations or flutters in chest • Constipation • Heaviness in chest

The physical within the emotional

I once had a patient who came to see me for a persistent low-grade cough. It was worse at night and seemed to subside during the day. She appeared to not have too many other stand-out symptoms but had hoped I'd be able to give her some relief as she found it frustrating. After several treatments, I realised I was getting nowhere. During her next appointment I decided to dig a little deeper to see if I could work out what I was missing. Knowing I had ticked all the boxes of treating her physical issue meant I could confidently turn to looking towards the emotions as being a possible cause, and so I asked her if she had any unresolved grief. Her answer held the clues I'd been searching for. She went on to tell me that after the passing of her mother, many years before, she had never actually cried or properly grieved her loss. She had pushed away her feelings enough times for them to appear to be gone, but as I see so often, they don't just magically melt away. It's not until they are actually acknowledged, felt and experienced that the physical symptoms leave too. I treated her accordingly and gave her a little pre-treatment warning that she might feel particularly low after her acupuncture treatment – after all, it was my intention to treat her on an emotional level rather than physical. I called to check in with her the following day, she called me a couple of names (all in the name of love) and shared with me that she had been crying for 24 hours straight, felt like total rubbish but knew it was for her health and her soul. By the time I saw her next, her cough was gone.

According to research performed by the department of physiology at the Showa University School of Medicine, Tokyo, Japan, respiration is important in maintaining physiological homeostasis and co-exists with emotions.

STRESS AND WHERE IT MANIFESTS IN YOUR BODY

- **Brain** – low mood, poor concentration, personality disorders
- **Hair** – hair loss, dry, brittle and for some oily hair
- **Mouth** – ulcers or cold sores can be induced by stress
- **Skin** – eczema, psoriasis, rashes and acne
- **Muscles** – muscle tension, muscle pain, twitches – all from stored emotions
- **Lungs** – coughing, wheezing and exacerbation of asthma or bronchitis
- **Heart** – palpitations, tightness in the chest, anxiety and excess stress from increased stress hormones can also raise blood pressure.
- **Digestive system** – under stress the digestive system shuts down as blood moves away to focus on other priorities, leading to gut issues, bowel troubles, etc.
- **Reproductive system** – delayed periods, inflammation leading to period pain, PMS and also bloating due to hormone imbalance.

THE 90-SECOND RULE

Some experts suggest that emotions last for various amounts of time. Those such as happiness or boredom tend to be more fleeting as opposed to those that are more deeply felt, such as sadness, frustration, worry or fear. Joan Rosenberg in her 2016 TED talk 'Emotional Mastery: The Gifted Wisdom of Unpleasant Feelings' suggests that feelings last on average for around 90 seconds. Just 90 seconds of riding it out, whatever it may be, and you will live through it. But no matter how many seconds it takes, when an emotion is fully embraced, it is more likely to last moments, not days. It's when we don't fully feel and embrace it that it can beat on and on like an unforgiving child throwing an epic tantrum in our overactive mind – sometimes this may last forever if we don't do something about it. Don't know about you, but the idea of a constant screaming sound in my head isn't appealing at all. Pass me the hot pins to poke in my eyeballs! Yet for many of us, unless we have this understanding, we choose it over feeling better because we know no different. And that's nobody's fault – we don't know what we don't know. We can feel it in parts of our body that we never knew possible and it can linger until we do something about it. Maybe you've made the connection when, after hearing bad news, you've felt sick to your stomach or perhaps you've been excited and felt it bound through your chest like nobody's business. We feel things not only on a physical level but equally on an emotional level too. TCM subscribes to the view that when we look at the organs for disharmony or illness, 50% of the treatment should be physical and the other 50% emotional.

> Just 90 seconds of riding it out, whatever it
> may be, and you will live through it.

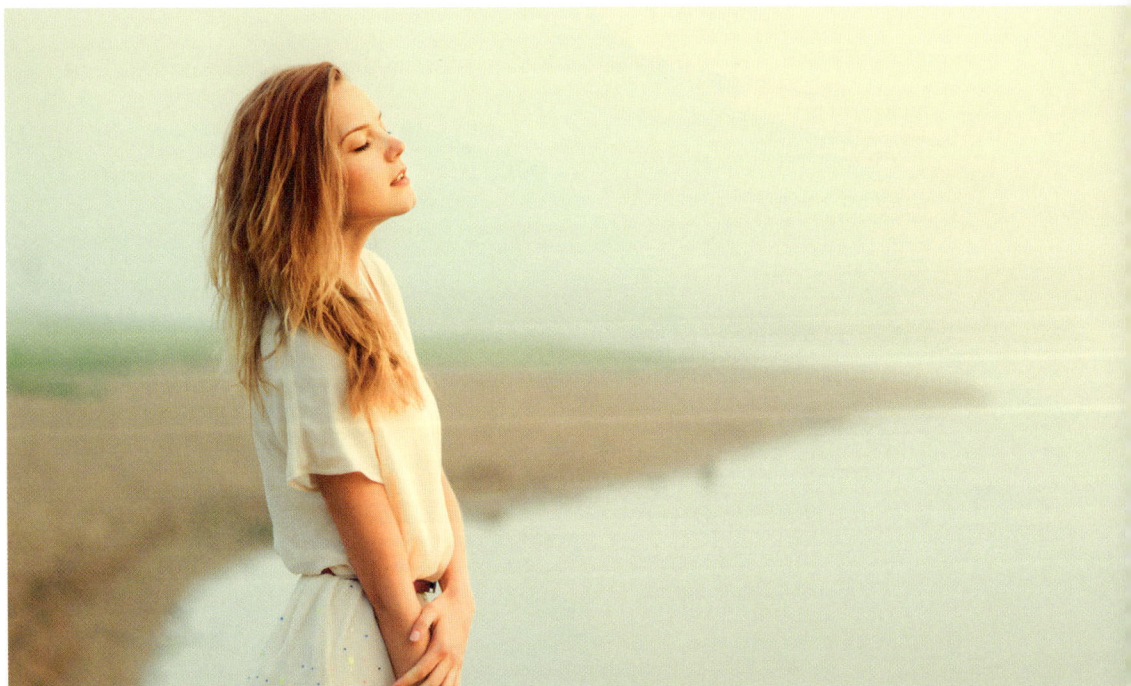

EMOTIONAL HEALTH PLAYS A PART IN PHYSICAL ILLNESS

More than ten years ago I was introduced to a process known as 'The Journey', developed by Brandon Bays, a motivational speaker and author who at the age of 39 discovered she had a tumour the size of a basketball growing in her stomach. It was through this time she was forced to look inwards and face up to her old emotional scars and wounds, which unlocked a very different approach to recovery, so profound in fact that the tumour was resolved in less than 7 weeks – something she was told was impossible. The premise behind what Brandon has gone on to teach thousands of people worldwide is the notion that cells in our body store memories which manifest as illness. This does not mean, of course, that you exclude the care of your doctor or specialist for physical or medical treatment of cancer; what Brandon tapped into was this emotional side to poor health – something that is still not fully understood from a Western medical perspective.

I was so drawn to this work after the birth of my daughter, Olivia, because it was a stand-out treatment that had immediate results in not only addressing my physical illness but my emotional health, too. Prior to learning of 'The Journey', I began to notice rather rapidly a hefty load of guilt that sat on my chest wherever I'd go. The fact was, there was no real reason for me to feel guilty. I had a wonderfully supportive husband, a business I was extremely proud of and I was almost 100% sure I didn't steal Olivia from the hospital (we'll save the birth story for another day). I had nothing to feel guilty about. As if carrying a heavy nappy bag around wasn't enough, I was carrying the weight of guilt around, too. So eventually I sought help, digging deeper into this idea that our emotions could manifest physically as my health continued to be less than average.

When it came to doing the work or the process of 'The Journey', I was guided by a facilitator who was able to take me back into my subconscious (that part of your brain you're not so privy to) to the first time I had felt this intense emotion of guilt, through a series of steps taking me back to that place of my younger self. What was revealed to me was nothing short of incredible. Through a series of guided processes I learnt the following:

I. The first time I'd felt this feeling was after my grandma had passed away; I was 10.

2. It all came back to a childhood experience (and ongoing subconscious memory) at my uncle's wedding. My grandmother had been terminally ill, all in the lead-up to the wedding, and I knew she was very sick and the emotions of this had built up considerably.

3. At the wedding my grandmother was in fabulous spirits and I, as a 10-year-old, was completely chuffed – all of a sudden, to me, she looked like she was feeling better and everybody was happy as they celebrated.

4. That night, as a 10-year-old girl, I made a promise to myself that I'd make sure everybody stayed happy from this moment on, no matter what cost. Of course, as a grown woman, I have the understanding that this wasn't at all possible, but as a child it was totally logical and so I made it my responsibility.

5. Several weeks later, my grandmother passed away and I was left feeling extremely guilty that I had failed and not lived up to my promise that I had made to my family and myself.

Now you and I know that as a logical person, there was no way I could have done what I set out to do that night, but as a 10-year-old girl, it seemed completely rational. Also, at that age, I didn't have the skills or the tools to deal with what I was experiencing and so I tucked those emotions that came along out of the way, reserved for another day. I could never have known that 'another day' was 20 years later. My emotions manifested into something that eventually became so big I had no choice but to deal with them.

Through this process, the first step is to identify what the moment or the cause of the feeling may have been, and the second part is to integrate the now new thought process into that moment, allowing the logical mind to change the internal story. This combination is a powerful winner in really getting to the root of many problems.

What I learnt with my 'Journey' practitioner completely intrigued me and I went on to study this practice in detail. Still to this day I'm so grateful for the experience and talk a lot about the process with patients to help them move through stuck emotions or childhood trauma or issues. The less time they have to sit and bubble, the sooner we can live the lives we were born to enjoy.

> Make sure that if you engage with someone to work through emotions or trauma that they have the appropriate professional qualifications to support you best.

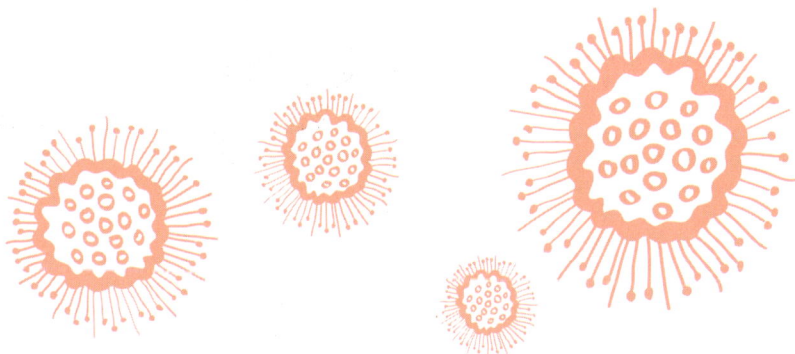

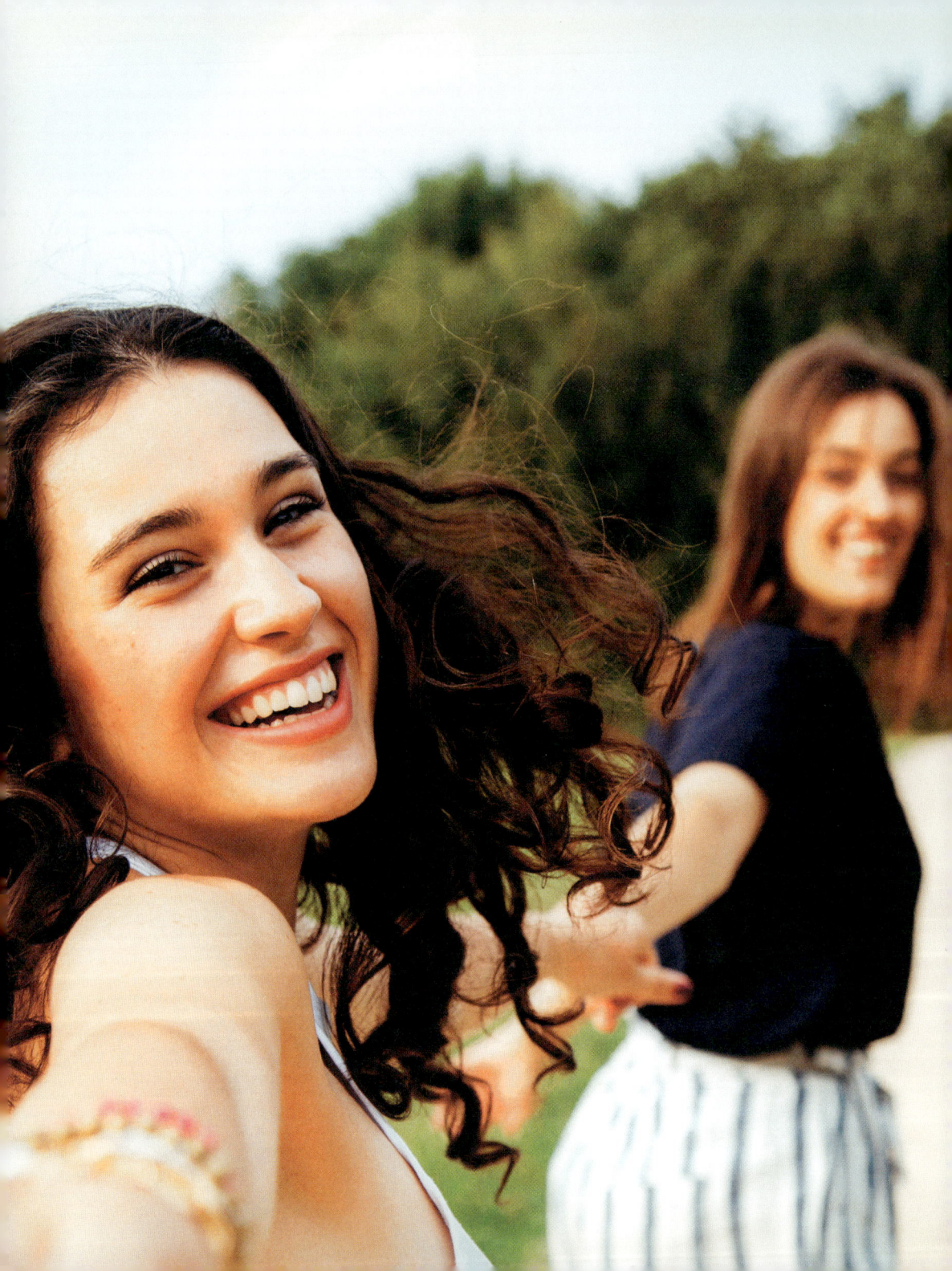

WORKSHEET: **USING EMOTIONS TO GET WHAT YOU WANT**

Have you ever experienced a true problem that turned out to be the best thing that ever happened to you? What if that problem was actually a catalyst to help you get what you want in life? Here's a practice I love to do when I have an issue.

1. Got a problem? Write it down.

_____

2. Ask yourself, where in your body do you feel it? (This may tell you a little more about what's going on internally if it is the same place constantly.)

_____

3. What would be the best possible outcome you could imagine if nothing could stop you from getting it? Write it down.

_____

4. What if this problem was put here to help you get exactly what you wanted in life but it was about tapping into how you feel, not how you don't want to feel? What would it feel like to have what you wanted? Write down these feelings.

_____

These feelings are your slipstream towards getting what you want.
Write them somewhere you can see them easily. When you're feeling
overwhelmed, upset or angry, see if you can recall these feelings instead.
It might take a little time but the practice is totally like any habit.
The more you practise, the more you gain access to what you want.

> '**Whether you think you can or think you can't, you're right.**' HENRY FORD

THE OBSERVER EFFECT

Perhaps you've met somebody who uses the phrase 'I'm just so sick and tired of xyz ...' Have you noticed anything about them? I bet my last dollar that they are constantly sick and always tired! It's not surprising at all, if we believe 'what we tell ourselves is what we create'. We are very powerful in making stuff happen, even though we might not yet realise this. I love author Pam Grout's picture she paints to explain this very idea of quantum physics. She explains that like radio signals, our thoughts broadcast our beliefs and expectations out into the big wide world. According to Pam, quantum physicists have proven that it is impossible for us to look at anything without impacting the thing we are looking at. It's referred to as the observer effect. There was an experiment known as Emoto's Water Experiment (by Dr Masaru Emoto) where the influence of words, thoughts, prayers, environment and music was measured on the crystalline structure of water to observe exactly how we can impact our surroundings by these factors. They exposed glasses of water to music, words, some they prayed over and others they changed the environment of where the glasses of water were located. The glasses of water that received positive or uplifting music, intentions or affirmations, when observed under magnification, were nothing short of breathtakingly beautiful. The opposite occurred in the glasses that received spoken words of hate and disgust, or sad or jarring music such as heavy metal. The droplets under magnification were not appealing to look at but more so looked like messy masses of confused crystals.

This tells us that when we focus our thoughts on the good stuff - like love, peace and possibility - your life experience will look exactly like this, filled with love and potential. But if your internal radio is tuned in to 'life is a trash can and it's all bad', this soundtrack is full of pain and suffering, and nobody needs to suffer unnecessarily. But worse still, you're literally feeding yourself trash with such a mindset. You actually have the remote to change the station - all it takes is pressing a few buttons, selecting what you want and away you go.

I know - it seems too good to be true and possibly overwhelming that I (or you) could be responsible for everything that can happen from here on (and actually have been for everything that has previously been). Of course, you aren't responsible for where you live or whom you were born to but we are responsible for how we approach this - there are some amazing people who come from hardship because of this. What if you could impact your ability to study, to get good grades and to get what you want in life? If we tap into this, can you see that the potential of amazingness is right there for you to sweep up and totally rock life with? You have this - we all do - it's just a matter of knowing how.

A Norwegian study in 2005 analysed a group of students right before they headed into an exam. The study group of students were prompted to draw on this positive way of thinking and, as they passed through the doors into the examination room, they told themselves, 'I can solve this task' and took their seat ready to rock the examination paper. The second group stated, 'I'm worried and will have problems solving other tasks too.' Something remarkable was found. The students who fed themselves this positive mind food had substantially less stress, and those who spoke negatively experienced their stress levels rise. It's a wonderful example of how our mindset influences our reality.

Harnessing your internal GPS

You might be shocked to understand that according to many cognitive neuroscientists, 95% of your thoughts are actually unconscious – that is, you don't really know you are thinking them. They are in the back of our mind, nattering away in every single moment of every day like an annoying younger brother or sister. Sometimes, they come to the front of our mind and we get a snapshot of awareness, but for the most part, we don't even know we are thinking them. We drown them out. Given we aren't necessarily privy to these thoughts (kinda rude considering they are in our own brain!) they can be harmful and unkind, all because we will take on things that we experience in life and create some type of internal dialogue around it.

What we must come to recognise is that we hold the power to influence each moment and we absolutely have a choice. Better still, when we make the wrong decision, we can decide to choose again. Maybe you've been faced with a curly choice, one that's had you torn in two. Perhaps you've made a decision, and while it has been the toughest call to date, it felt so darn right that you just knew it had to be that way. But on the flip side, maybe you made a decision that was the safe choice, or conversely a risky choice, and immediately you knew it wasn't right. From the pit of your stomach you knew that you'd made the wrong decision. Tapping into our intuition or our gut feeling can be the biggest gift once we learn to nurture it, ultimately because it is never, ever wrong. It is like your very own internal tracking device that allows you to hone in on what works for you. The trick in this is remembering that it actually only works for you and nobody else, since nobody else is you.

Your intuition is like your own internal device that allows you to know what's right for you.

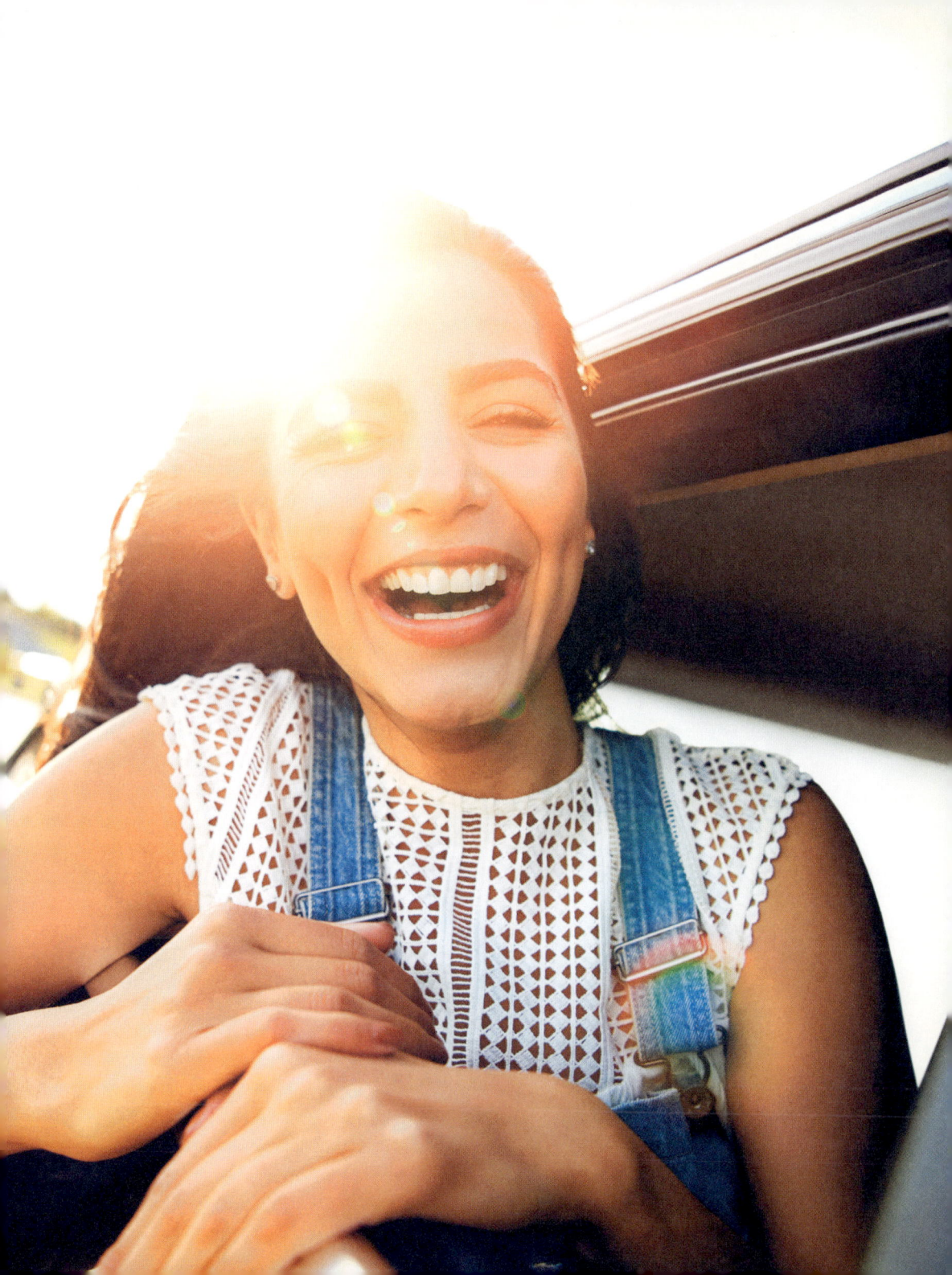

Some refer to your intuition as your sixth sense or gut feeling. It's not too difficult to zone into your gut feeling, although when your body is in disharmony, such as in times of hormone imbalance, it can be a little tricky. But as you learn to apply the goodness of this book, it will become clearer and easier.

I suggest starting with an issue that isn't too life changing to begin with, say perhaps something like making a choice of going out or staying in. Think deeply about what your body is telling you. Perhaps you're feeling good and there's a strong need to be social and hang out with friends. But equally your body might be asking for some self care and staying in is the option you're drawn to, even though your best friend is begging for you to chaperone her. There is no external right or wrong (though I'm not saying do anything illegal or that would harm someone!); there is just your own internal wellbeing and living that count most.

> Allow your gut to guide you – it's like your very own internal GPS device.

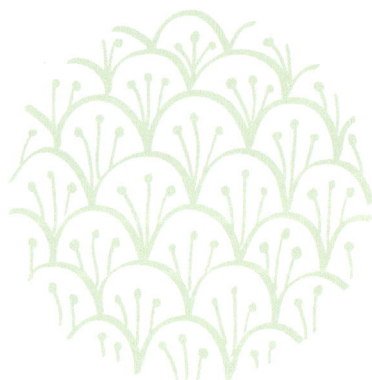

WORKSHEET: **HOW TO WORK THROUGH DECISIONS**

When do you need to make the choice by?

What would be the best-case scenario?

What would be the worst-case scenario?

What does your intuition tell you?

What are you choosing?

What is your plan?

Almost all of the time, what felt like a tough decision today was actually an amazing experience and created room for change and growth. Can you think back to a time where you had to make a tough call and it propelled you to your next level of greatness? We don't necessarily need to feel stressed or overwhelmed, we just need to remind ourselves that choice creates change and it always works out. AND pain or emotion lasts no longer than 90 seconds when we embrace it fully. Moving forward is key. Getting stuck can be an easy choice, but it keeps us in a perpetual state of limbo and often excess pain. Nobody needs to live in limbo any longer!

CHAPTER 3

Your body changes

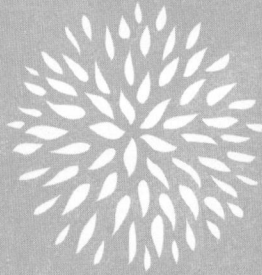

'Two basic rules of life are:
1) Change is inevitable.
2) Everybody resists change.'

W. EDWARDS DEMING

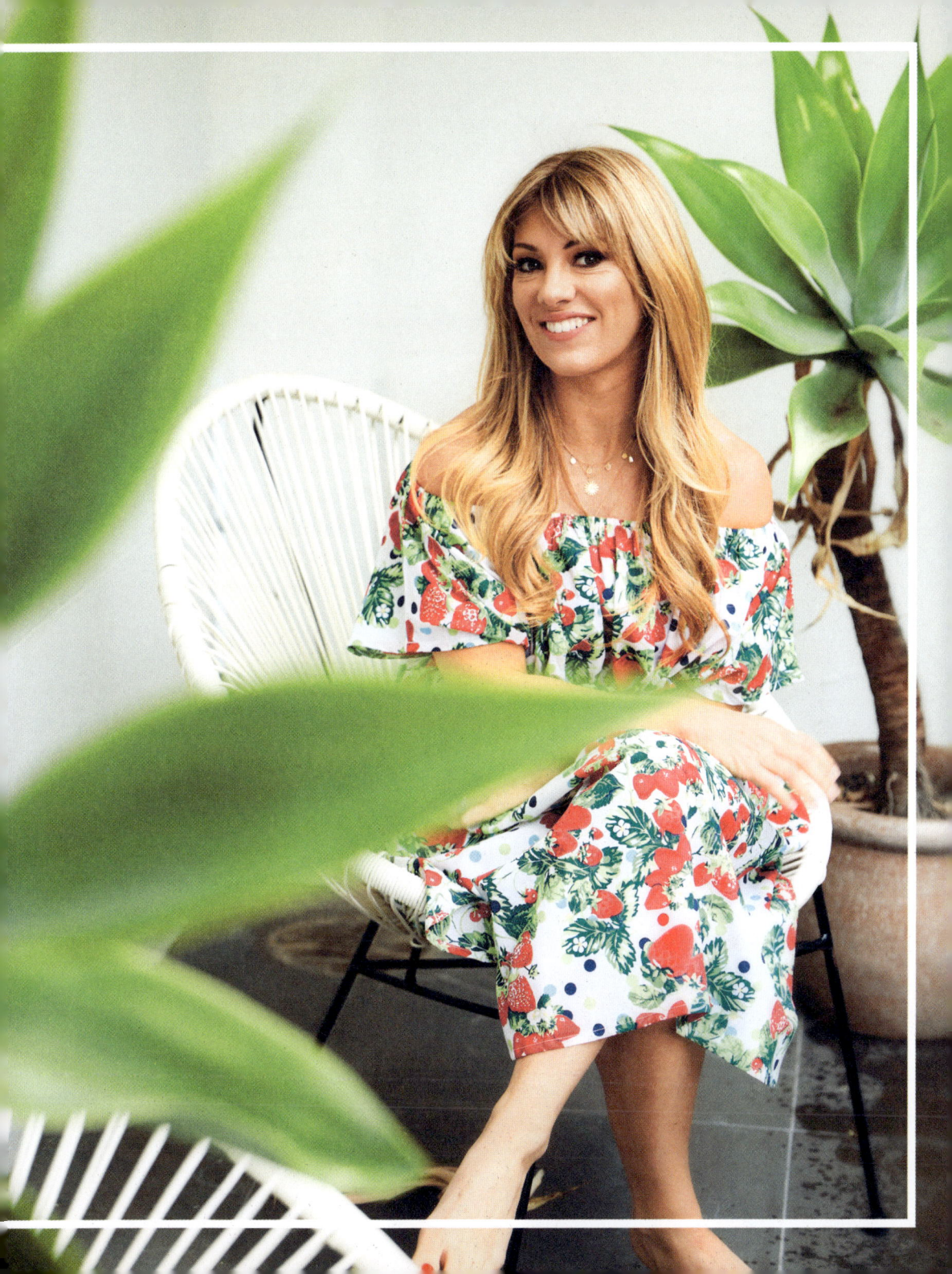

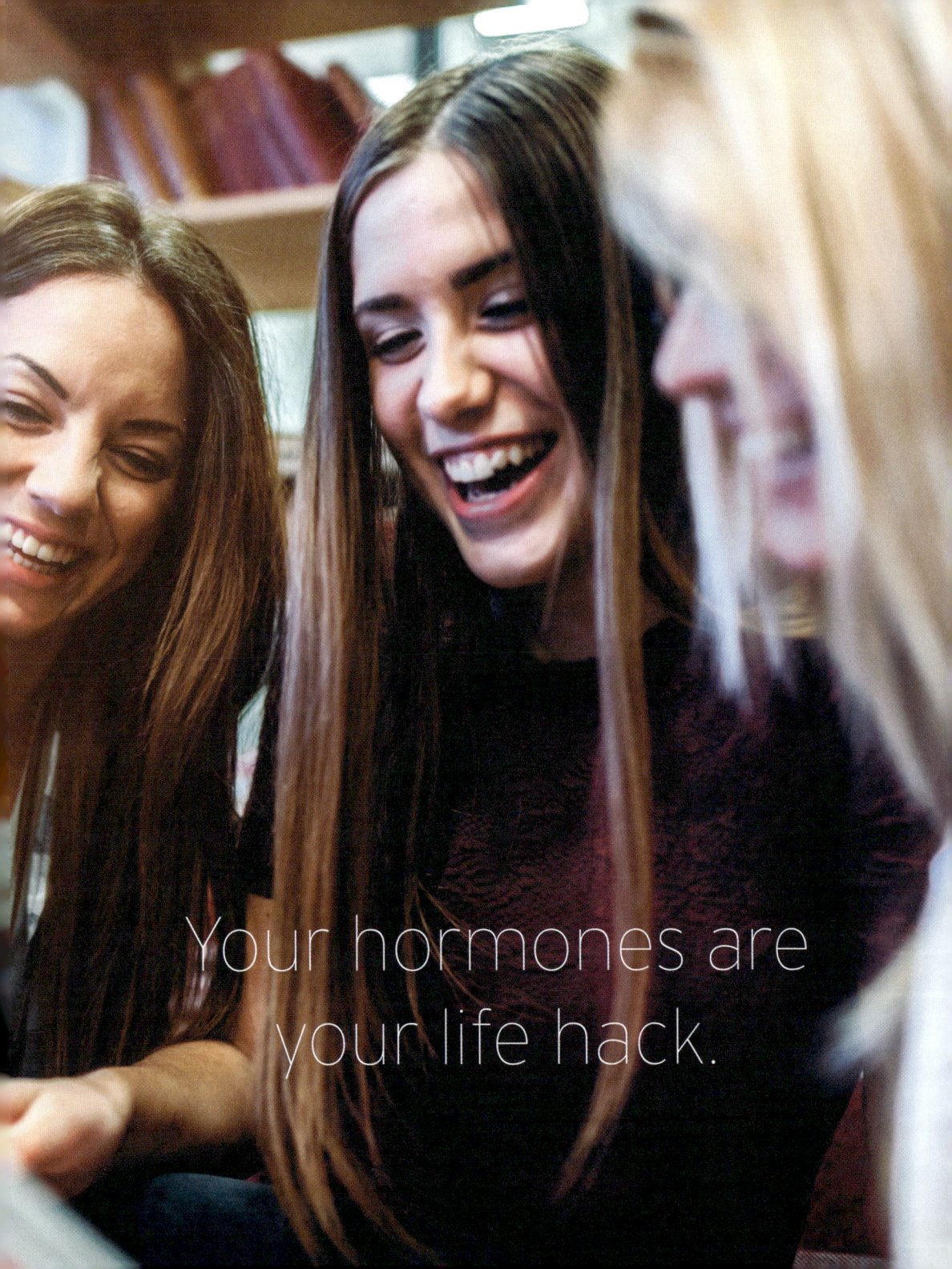

Your hormones are
your life hack.

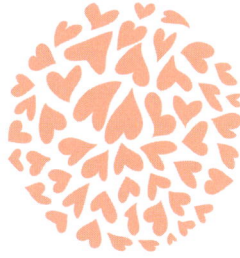

Playing detective – using your symptoms as your clues

YOU WILL LEARN:

• what your symptoms are telling you

• all about hormone cycles, what happens and when

Change is important yet we often resist it because it feels so darn scary. We can retaliate, hold our own pity party, tantrum out and stomp our feet, but try as we might, we can't stop the world from turning or pull the brake on the calendar ticking over. It appears we've become really good at fearing the unknown and pushing mighty hard against it.

Over time I've come to learn that **the biggest gift we can give ourselves is education.** When we understand something, we no longer approach it from fear or anxiety, and best of all we can take back our own power and not be at the mercy of others who don't in fact live in the skin we're in. We can make informed choices that serve us; we ask questions, get the facts and feel empowered. It becomes a very secure place to operate from and if you can couple this with your new-found intuition to guide you, it's a recipe for amazing success. And while your body may change in wild and wonderful ways, one thing is for sure: change is going to happen so let's learn to embrace it.

Our bodies are certainly cyclic and Traditional Chinese Medicine beautifully summarises these cycles for women to come around every seven to eight years or so. This said, it is interesting to observe that young women are finding the onset of their periods happening earlier and earlier. It was once considered that around 11 years of age was the average age the period would show up but it appears to be shifting even earlier in recent years. There are several reasons for this, and various studies have been done looking into the reasons why this may be happening. Here are some possible reasons.

• Excess oestrogen via the diet. Oestrogen can be driven wild by other factors that mimic oestrogen, including excess consumption of soy, non-organic meats as well as environmental factors like exposure to electromagnetic fields and chemicals in our personal care products and cleaning products.

• Over-consumption of processed foods such as soft drinks and fried foods may contribute to excess weight gain. Oestrogen is an anabolic hormone and as we learnt it is mostly made by the ovaries; however, it is also excreted from our fat cells. One study concluded that consumption of sugary drinks was positively associated with early onset of the period and possibly linked to an increase in PCOS.

A NOTE ON SOY.

Soy isn't supposed to be a meal replacement and when we look at how it is traditionally prepared and consumed, it is done so alongside meat and vegetables - not as a stand-alone 'food group'. Soy is also highly processed and it has made its way into many foods because it is an excellent thickener; some of us have also used it as an alternative to dairy. Soy is fine to enjoy sporadically, like any other legume, but when it becomes an inclusion at almost every meal, it may be a problem for your hormones. The effects will vary from person to person. With this in mind, it is best to leave it on the lower consumption list - definitely no more than one serve every few days or so.

• Stress drives oestrogen crazy and pushes all the right buttons to see it climb high. We live at a time where stress is a modern-day epidemic. Lucky for you, I've got loads of tools to help! And for more information, head to my stress course on www.debunkingstress.com.

Early onset of the menses (aka your period) is something to keep an eye on. Perhaps yours showed up early and you thought nothing of it. If you're in this camp, it's important to look at your oestrogen levels and to adopt some of the principles in this book to take better control of your hormones. Excess oestrogen can become a pesky issue that comes with a boot-full of symptoms, and over time can be at the core of some pretty nasty illnesses. It is believed that women who get their period earlier than average are at a greater risk of breast cancer later on in life. This isn't anything to lose your cool over, but it is valuable information to make some changes now to set you up for the long haul because it can often be easily managed. We're still learning in this area, but what this effectively means is that if you have a predisposition towards oestrogen-related conditions, you can implement strategies to lessen the impact. Now that you know this, it can be excellent motivation to ensure that your hormones are always a priority for you and your long-term health.

Now why am I telling you this? You most probably do not have menopause on your radar (although maybe you can help educate your mum or your much-loved elders in your life), and you are not likely to be ready to go forward and create your very own football team of tiny humans. I'm telling you this because what you do at each and every stage of your life affects the next stage, yet we often focus only on what is happening here and now.

What you do at each and every stage of your life affects the next – hoping it will get better isn't enough.

Take the previous example of excess oestrogen and breast cancer. Knowing these small snippets of information can literally save our lives in years to come. While it might feel nice to live it up and not worry about things until there is actually a real issue, the fact is, not only should we be thinking about long-term health, we must. What's more, we don't 'arrive' at illness down the track far into the future, it's literally the accumulation of everything we've done up until the point of diagnosis that has taken health in a direction we may not want. Each and every phase of your life has a purpose and is essential for us to move into the next. We can't go from first to home base, as skipping two bases would show up with a magnitude of symptoms and you'd miss all the adaptations your body makes along the way. Change is everything and working with your flow is essential. **It's therefore vital that we establish something right here and now. Your unwanted symptoms are simply clues into your internal environment.**

THE 8-YEAR CYCLES OF HORMONES ACCORDING TO TCM

BY 8 YEARS OF AGE:

We commence puberty. Young girls begin to show breast buds and there may be changes with cervical fluid as they prepare for the arrival of the period. This doesn't mean the period arrives at 8; it tends to show up between 11 and 14 years on average but, as discussed, girls' periods are showing up earlier.

BY 16 YEARS OF AGE:

The menstrual cycle is establishing itself (yes, it's normal for it to be irregular, right up until you're 18-20). We go through a period of more hormone changes marked by weight gain (all normal) and possibly some pretty impressive emotions to match. Good news is, this is just a phase, too, and things do settle down ... eventually.

FROM 24 YEARS OF AGE:

We hit the prime of our fertility. We're baby ready, our cycles should be regular and we feel good, generally. Although modern lifestyle may encroach, things are mostly dandy.

FROM 32 YEARS OF AGE:

Women are still very fertile (contrary to what we're too often told) and generally have a better understanding of their hormones and cycles. From our mid 30s, our hormones begin to change (again). Perimenopause hits - this transition begins at 35.

As unruly as they may be, symptoms arise for a very good reason: to alert you that something odd is up. It's usually in response to some kind of load or stress, be it internal, external or emotional. This could result from a smorgasbord of underlying issues. I like to give my patients a checklist when they come into my clinic of all the contributing factors that may be showing up, causing havoc within the body. I do this as a means to show them the 'stressors' that could be running the show and to be able to shine a spotlight on the cause – rather than just treating symptoms alone. We can continue to treat symptoms, which of course may offer some short-term relief, but if we don't get to the crux of the issue, we may only ever be left chasing our tail. **Treating the cause is key.**

Here are my top 10 most common causes of hormone imbalance and unwanted symptoms.

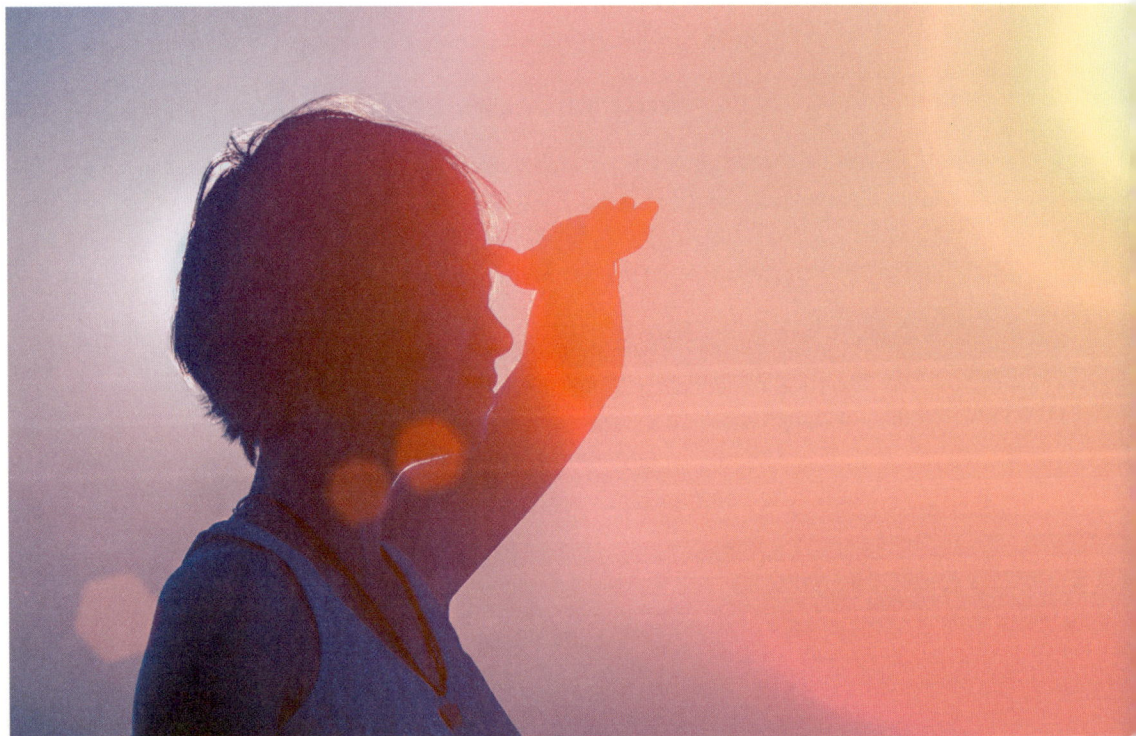

Common causes of hormone imbalance

1. Intolerances

Anything that you are intolerant to may place a huge amount of stress on your body, especially your digestive system. Intolerances come in all shapes and sizes, some more obvious than others. The main offenders include the delicious stuff (but not so great for your insides), gluten, sugar and dairy. These foods may be your tastebuds' foods of choice, but each and every time you consume them they send your digestive system into a state of panic. Be careful to fully understand what an intolerance is. It isn't an allergy – allergies generally are life threatening and can result in reactions that could be fatal, such as anaphylaxis. An intolerance is far less serious, although may still be driving your issues and causing you a considerable amount of discomfort. An intolerance is a food that, at this point in time, your body can't adequately digest. Other common offenders I see in the clinic are foods like eggs, nuts, tomatoes, onions and garlic, to name only a few of many. Once you make good inroads into gut health (we'll get into this), you should find yourself able to tolerate a range of foods; some in smaller quantities but you will be ok to consume them without too many issues.

2. Nutrient deficiencies

When the gut can't assimilate adequately, it may mean that we eventually begin to lack certain essential vitamins and minerals that are key for balanced health and happy hormones. The same goes for those with a poor diet. Dr Tom O'Bryan (a specialist in non-celiac gluten sensitivity) once said to me in a podcast that food is either of benefit or deficit. It either nourishes your body or depletes it. These words have rung in my brain ever since, almost every time I make a food choice. Ask yourself, is your plate going to give your body everything it needs or make you double over in pain? You can't skimp on food. It's simply just not one of those things you can cut corners with.

3. Poor gut function, the microbiome and inflammation

Your gut is the epicentre of your entire being. It not only digests your food but it shapes around 80% of your immune function, as well as being your emotion centre. Research now tells us that the microbiome – that is, the constellation of bacteria that live in us and on us – contains genes that influence how our own genes work. Scientists from the Babraham Institute in the UK discovered that DNA in the epithelial tissues (i.e. the wall) of the colon contain chemicals known to act as an epigenetic switch, turning genes on and off! Epigenetics refers to the external environment which changes how our genes behave, not the actual changes to the genes which influence how they work.

When the gut flora is compromised by the use of antibiotics or medications such as the oral contraceptive pill, the gut wall itself becomes vulnerable. For the gut to be happy, it relies on two things to be sound – the permeability and the microbiome. If there is overgrowth of unhealthy or unwanted bacteria OR complete eradication of this bacteria, the right signals for optimal body function aren't necessarily activated or signalled. We generally can restore good bacteria with probiotic foods (such as kombucha or fermented vegetables like sauerkraut) as well as by eliminating certain stressful or taxing foods (such as sugar, gluten and dairy) that overwhelm the gut or cause overgrowth of the unwanted bacteria.

The gut permeability relies on the cell junctions that make up the wall of the digestive system being nice and tightly packed together. When there are gaps between the junctions or they are compromised, food can 'leak' out of the gut, causing inflammation and triggering an autoimmune response. This is known as leaky gut. You may have heard the term before and the name says it all. When the gut is 'leaky', overtime, small gaps between the cells or holes allow waste and toxins to escape and move into the bloodstream. For a great illustration of a leaky gut, see Chapter 5.

When food begins to leak out of the digestive system it can cause a plethora of issues, including inflammation, and can trigger other responses in the body like autoimmune issues. This can show up in a varied number of ways. The factor that dictates this most is your genes. It may explain why you have endometriosis but your friend doesn't. But don't think she is exempt, it may show up somewhere else for her like eczema or acne. By focusing on the gut you can make mammoth inroads to your health and wellbeing. In fact, for most patients, we must start here. You may wonder if you can ever 'fix' leaky gut, and the reality is that we are at risk of unfavourable gut health if we don't care for ourselves, no less than if we are deficient in certain vitamins and minerals. If we don't look after ourselves properly, we can suffer. It comes down to what I call 'the everyday effect'; that is, what you do each and every single day is what counts most. Gut health is a work in progress – ensuring that you are doing your best each and every day will allow your body to perform optimally.

The gut–hormone connection is where certain bacteria strains assist in the metabolism of various influences, for example, oestrogen. Those gut bacteria specific to oestrogen have been named estrobolome. Estrobolome metabolises oestrogen. We're not yet at a stage of being able to implant specific strains of bacteria, so our focus is more on working on the gut as a whole to re-colonise the beneficial strains of bacteria. We talk more about how we can get this back on track in the following chapters.

4. Emotional wellbeing

You may be shocked to learn that your emotional health is what I would call the biggest influence on your overall wellbeing. You may tick every physical box when it comes to your health: you have an amazing diet, healthy sleep and great sleep hygiene, you exercise regularly and keep things in check where possible. However, if your mindset is off, every single cell in your body knows – it's like big brother is talking. One of my favourite sayings states, **'Be careful what you think, every cell in your body is eavesdropping'.**

As we've learnt, your cellular activity is always responding to the external environment. It's always important to have this on your radar. For some of us, there has been known trauma like an accident or a childhood incident that may fuel our emotional health. For others, it may be a mystery what the root cause here is, however, it must always be considered and there are a variety of sneaky ways we can dig in deeper to the depths of our subconscious. As we learnt in Chapter 2, it's about working out where this stems from.

5. Detoxification

The word 'detox' gets thrown around like confetti, often getting a bad rap because of some kind of gruelling regime that must be adhered to like super glue to get results. We're not talking about diving into a 'detoxification process' that involves little more than air and lemon juice. Such regimens can be a disaster for your hormones – I don't advocate for these at all. I want you to be acquainted with your liver. In a ship-shape world, we wouldn't need to cleanse the body, it actually does a pretty good job of it on its own; however, there can be certain factors (you guessed it, 'stressors') that impact your body's detoxification ability and in our modern lives these factors add up and have their way with our internal workings. There are many organs involved in the process of detoxification. I tend to start with looking at the gut and the liver when it comes to the first steps on the ladder, and the kidneys aren't too far behind. Your liver is responsible for the detoxification of testosterone and oestrogen and, for many, this can be at the core of their hormone imbalance, should this not be in check.

There are a few very simple steps (listed on the following pages) you can implement to have your liver on its way to happier days that don't involve you sipping on air through a straw with a bit of pepper thrown in. We'll be digging deeper into this in the coming pages.

6. Environment

We are each a product of our own environment – yet again, our cells are responsive to what goes on around us. If you live in a messy space, your health may very well pick up on it. A temporarily dishevelled bedroom of course won't necessarily do any harm, but the long-term exposure to toxins in our environment, poor air quality, chemicals, mould and other toxic factors can certainly affect us – and some more than others. What affects you and why certainly is genetic, but it's all about finding the clues. Bottom line, keep your surroundings tidy and in check. That alone may not be the solution to your health issues but it sure is an easy fix that generally can be done with ease (unless you are a long-term hoarder).

7. Hidden infections

It's tricky for us to sometimes really know exactly what's going on in that internal landscape. When things aren't moving along nicely it may be a result of a pesky hidden infection or bug that's really never taken its eviction notice seriously. This can be a result of a virus, such as glandular fever, or exposure to something on an exotic trip to the middle of the Amazon. Whatever the reason, it's always good to have it checked out.

A WORD ON STIs ...

I'll never forget my first opportunity to sit in on a laparoscopy (exploratory surgery of the lower abdomen, mostly reserved for gynecological issues and very common when there's suspected endometriosis or adenomyosis) where the gynecologist performing surgery boldly announced, 'Oh gosh, close this woman up, she's full of chlamydia!' Her disease had affected her fertility. It was so sad to think that having unprotected sex when she was younger affected her fertility in her 30s. Vaginal infections are not necessarily STIs (Sexually Transmitted Infections). However, there are a host of issues that can arise with infections and inflammation of the vagina, discussed further in Chapter 8. But to summarise: Vaginitis is a name given to a host of inflammatory conditions including bacterial vaginosis and candida as well as other issues such as genital warts and herpes. STIs include chlamydia, gonorrhea and trichomoniasis, which are all common. Bottom line: If you are sexually active, use a condom or appropriate barrier method (discussed in Chapter 6).

8. Toxin exposure

Chemicals are all around us and can be darn difficult to escape. Our body products, shampoos and conditioners, washing detergents, cleaning materials, sprays on our fruit and vegetables or nasties in our water all make their way into our body and affect us – like it or not. The trick is not to sweat the small stuff; however, making changes that are simple and easy do count. While it's probably not possible for you to walk around with your very own air purifier strapped to your forehead, there are some very simple fixes to improve your external environment where it matters most – at home. Switching to non-chemical products is a very easy step in the right direction.

For many, by the time we leave the house in the morning we may have exposed ourselves to around 80 chemicals, all from the 7 or 8 personal hygiene products we use as staples in our morning routine. We may have washed our body and our hair, styled our hair, applied makeup, deodorant and perfume, all before 9 am. This doesn't factor in any of the other small fixes like your tried-and-true acne ointment, rash cream or non-organic sanitary products. It's important you know what you are exposing yourself to. In fact, if you can't eat it, should you really put it on your body? Probably not (although I'm not advocating for eating tampons but you know what I mean!).

9. Poor stress response

Even when just a handful of the above factors are at play, the body is operating out of a state of heightened stress. But this is two pronged. Stress may be internal as a result of these deficiencies or disturbances we may find ourselves in the grips of, but it can also be a choice. We begin to choose stress because our adrenals are in overdrive and it feels weirdly safe, even though our body may be screaming for another way. Stress is darn hard to get a handle on. But we've also adopted the crazy idea that if we aren't stressed, we can't be effective or get a job done well. We've married stress to success. Now, I'm all for happy partnerships but these two, stress and success, are not all they're cracked up to be. There is only so long one can operate in this hectic and toxic space, before things come crashing down.

Best news of all, for the most part we get to choose. Do we choose stress or do we choose ease? It doesn't make us any less successful if we don't buy into stress and its grips; in fact, on the contrary. Let's do less to achieve more – stay with me on this, I promise I will show you how.

IO. EMF exposure

Your favourite wifi source may be what you believe keeps you alive – maybe it's your lifeline. You might find the idea of disconnecting frightening! However, Electromagnetic Fields, or EMFs, can affect your health and your hormones. EMFs can cause a host of issues as they change the frequency of your brainwaves as your eyes stare at that blue-lit screen on your phone, computer or device. But don't sweat it (remember we're all on the ease train here); there are a few simple fixes that can make a profound impact.

HOW TO PROTECT YOUR HORMONES FROM BEING AFFECTED BY YOUR PHONE'S BLUE LIGHT

1. Turn off the blue light on your phone.

2. Avoid going to bed with your phone.

3. Shut down the wifi before bed.

4. Avoid bluetooth where you can.

Power down your wifi overnight. It may even help you avoid purchasing items online while you sleep ;)

SHOULD I USE A PAD OR A TAMPON?

It's a good question and one we may put way too much thought into because, as we've come to learn, we are all so different. Tampons come in a range of sizes, some with applicators and some without. The main point is to learn if you like using them or not but there really is no stress either way. Pads may be your best option when you first start to menstruate or for those with period pain (it's been suggested that tampons may contribute to period pain although there is no solid evidence to support this). Toxic Shock Syndrome (TSS) is said to be an issue if you leave a tampon in for too long (although this would possibly be for many hours, not just several), although I'm yet to find somebody who has suffered from this. Being hygienic is the most important aspect of health when it comes to pads and tampons – changing them regularly (as needed) tends to work best, approximately every 4 hours or so. But if you were to leave it in for a little longer, chances are you would be more than fine. Of course if you are concerned, always seek the right advice but TSS is a bacterial infection that you would tend to see fairly obviously and with a rapid onset of symptoms.

The use of menstrual cups has become something of the times – in my experience women either love them or hate them. The cup is placed inside much like a tampon but rather than absorbing, it collects the menstrual blood. If your tampon or cup is inserted correctly, you shouldn't be able to feel it. Again, there is no right or wrong. It comes down to preference and regardless of what you prefer, be it pad, tampon or cup, it may be a matter of it simply taking some time for you to get comfortable with them.

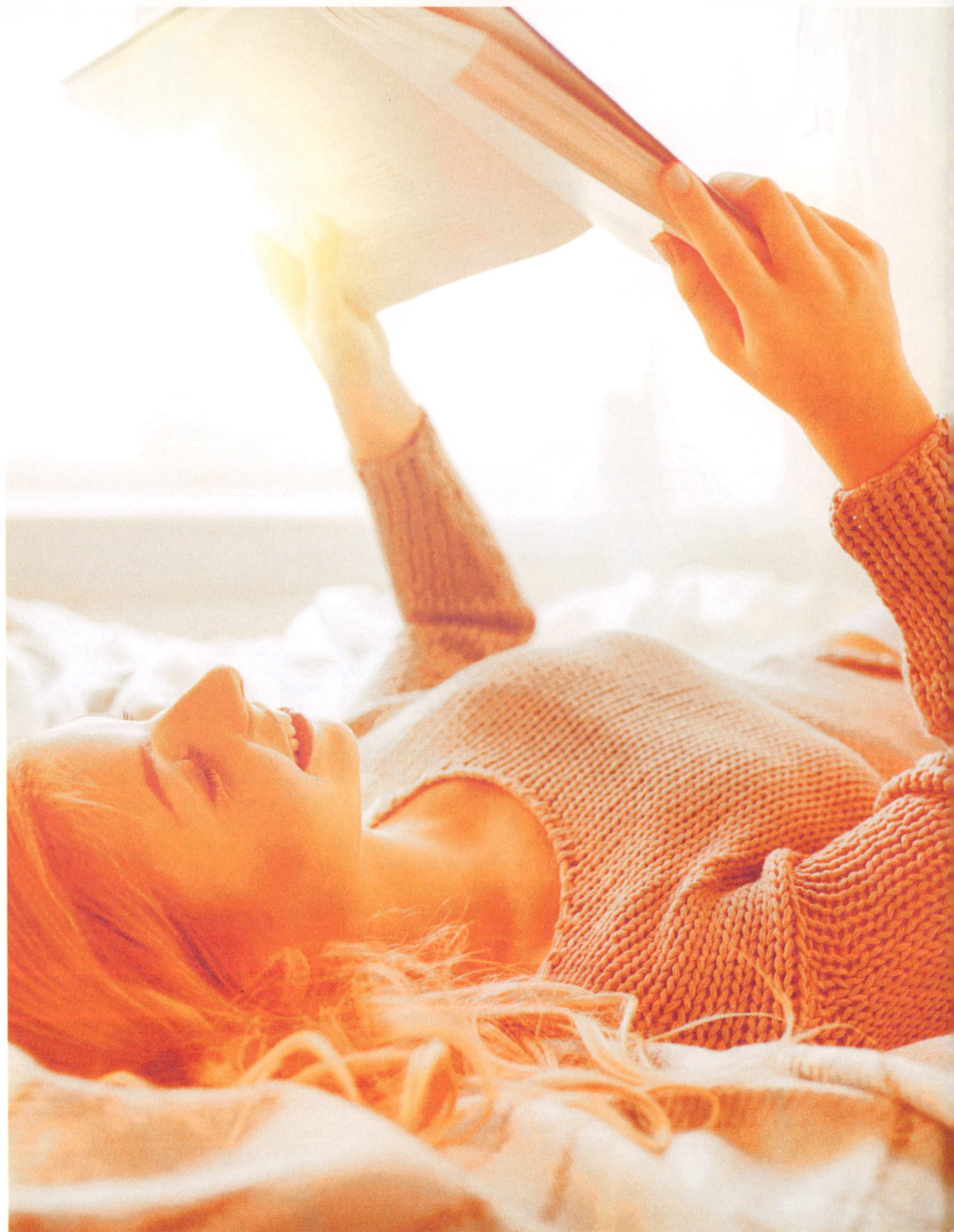

MAKING YOUR GENES BEHAVE

While our genes dictate what we may have been 'dealt', it's simply not acceptable to settle. Our genes are like our blueprint, but it is our epigenetics that are the sweet spot if we so want. Epigenetics is the term for how everything outside of our DNA can actually influence our genes – in this instance these 10 factors we've just discussed can encourage our genes to behave or misbehave. Just because you're predisposed (genetically speaking) doesn't mean you have to develop such conditions and symptoms. The trick is to look at your family history and begin decoding.

Aunt Nora's thyroid problem possibly indicates you too may have the same struggles if you don't switch the station. If your mum has endometriosis or Polycystic Ovarian Syndrome (PCOS), chances are you have that same potential and potential is the key word here. It doesn't have to happen but it may well do if you don't steer your health to its best. With a few tricks and lifestyle changes, we can keep symptoms at bay or at the very least assist you in managing them. The bottom line is just because your symptoms may be out of control doesn't mean that's it for you. There is a better way and this book will show you how. It's all about using the information that your body is literally spitting out at you and making some changes.

CHAPTER 4

Hormone imbalances

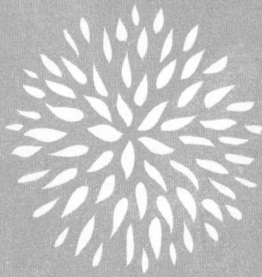

'Balance is not something you find, it's something you create.'

JANA KINGSFORD

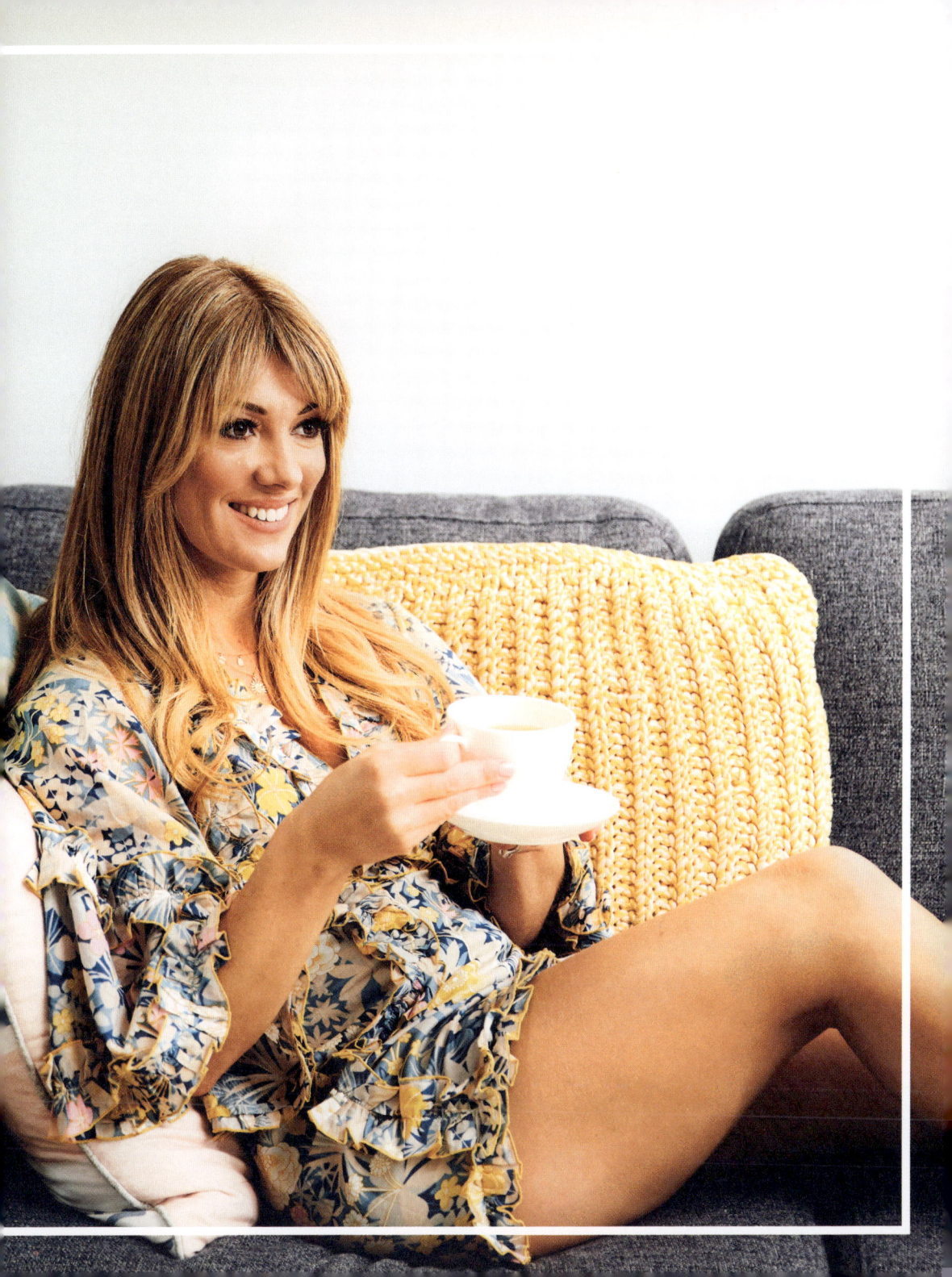

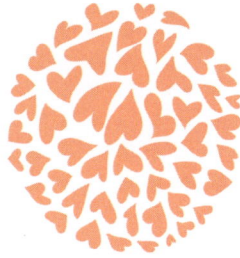

What goes up *can* come down

YOU WILL LEARN ABOUT:

• weight gain • acne • mood swings and PMS • bloating
• breast changes • changes 'down there' • PCOS
• endometriosis • painful periods • missing periods

Your body changes. Now that we know change is inevitable and pushing against it is like trying to apply fake lashes in the dark (totally impossible), we can start to get excited by the fact that our body is telling us each and every day specific signs and symptoms that help us to decode what's really going on.

Any changes you see provide deep clues, each specific to your own unique self; however, with a bit of guidance you may begin to really get to the core of what's actually causing your unwanted symptoms.

Weight gain

There can be many reasons why our weight can change, especially in our later teen years. Polycystic Ovarian Syndrome (PCOS) expert Dr Fiona McCollough shares how researchers now believe that as girls go through puberty, the hormone system very temporarily enters a state similar to that of PCOS. We discuss PCOS in greater detail in a moment. For most women, this weight gain passes. You may notice also as your breasts grow, your shape may too have changed. You're no longer 12 and you have hips to match. Who wants to be 12 forever anyway?

Often women are told if they just lose weight, their symptoms will resolve. We've become very fixated on weight but have lost track of what is healthy. Your healthy weight and your ideal weight may actually be miles apart and we are all put on this beautiful earth in all different shapes and sizes. As a general rule, what you weigh is not by choice (unless there are some pretty unhealthy eating patterns, which inevitably lead to a host of long-term complications). Your weight is therefore a direct result of genetics, hormones and neurotransmitters, and is substantially influenced by your childhood weight as well as how you see food and have learnt to consume it as a child. I struggled for years with that last mouthful on my plate. As a child, I was always told to eat every last mouthful or there would be no dessert. Now I know better and I trust you've learnt that too. Eating until satiated is extremely important but, as you will learn, wholefoods that tick nutritional boxes will allow us to feel full and satisfied. Empty calories, not so much. Hence why we can smash a packet of sweets and not feel sick.

Sugar is designed to be a momentary fuel source and it doesn't make us feel full.

Studies now show that once we have been a certain weight for a period of time, dieting may cause initial weight loss but it is almost certainly followed by weight gain. If you've found yourself overweight since you were a child, your metabolism works very differently from somebody who has been lean all their life, and the same regimen won't work because you are both built completely differently.

Healthy is the new lean and thank goodness! Given the factors that determine our weight are that of the metabolism, the gut, the thyroid and your hormones, the trick does not lie in what you deprive yourself of but more so what you can allow yourself in abundance. Rather than restrictions, ticking nutritional boxes is key and it's not as hard as we may think. The trick is getting the metabolism and hormones happy and I'm going to continue to show you how right here!

It's far better (and more effective for the long term) to move quickly towards your healthy and stable weight due to good nutrition than to yo-yo up and down between dress sizes. Diets generally cause more harm than good. We talk about what you put in your mouth and also about lifestyle. Plus, you've got to eat, so why not make it count.

In the pages that follow, you'll find a bunch of recipes that will help take you towards your healthier and brighter self. Food plays a huge role in health – in fact I think it is the most important. I can't wait for you to tag me in the recipes you create so I get to see your inner masterchef!

Feeling beautiful is your key to looking beautiful. Those two are a match made in heaven.

Acne

Your skin is your largest organ, but very often the most neglected. It's also important to understand that your skin absorbs up to 80% of what you apply topically - consider your skin a slipstream to your endocrine (hormone) system. The relationship with your gut health and your skin is very much intertwined, too. Your skin is one of the only ways (besides your mouth or your bowels) that your body is able to rid itself of toxins so when we see issues such as acne, eczema, psoriasis, dermatitis and rashes, the first place to start looking is at gut health.

Your skin is like a slipstream to your endocrine system.

We go through puberty sometime in our teen years, where as mentioned, researchers now believe that our body is 'temporarily' in PCOS mode, and along with this may come spots and dots. Acne can be extremely frustrating and often is a result of changing hormones; however, some can experience acne throughout their entire life. Increased levels of androgens (including testosterone) are often at the centre of most women's acne. These elevated levels of androgens increase the formation of comedones (whiteheads and blackheads) in the skin by increasing sebum production, which changes the skin cells. Bacteria accumulate and the end result of this is an increased number of pustules and papules (pimples) and blackheads, and nobody wants masses of either. We all want clear skin and the key to clear skin is honing in on why it's playing funny business in the first place.

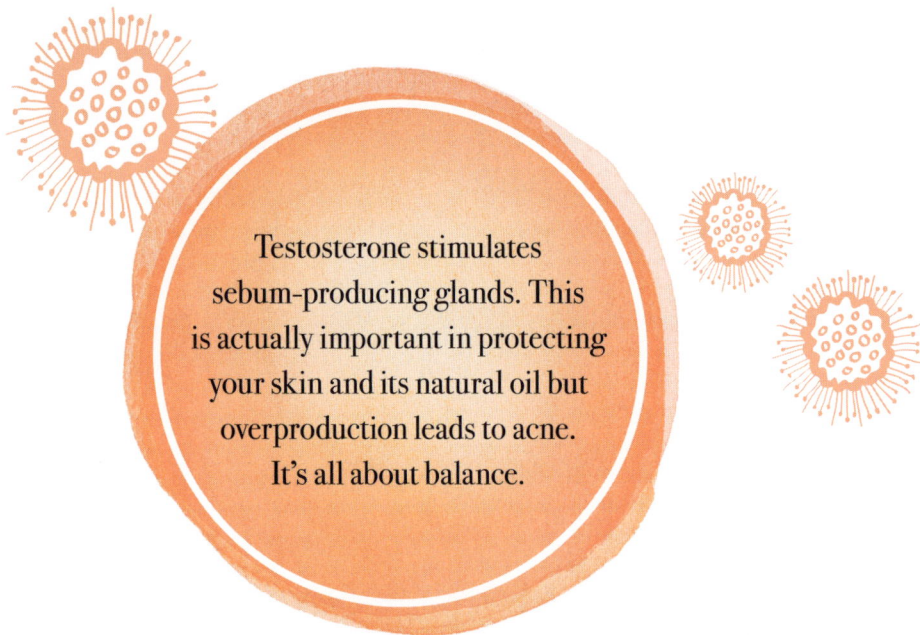

> Testosterone stimulates sebum-producing glands. This is actually important in protecting your skin and its natural oil but overproduction leads to acne. It's all about balance.

Where your acne accumulates tells you a few clues about what may be going on internally and gives you a window into the best means of treatment for your skin.

All of our major sex hormones (oestrogen, progesterone and testosterone) are important for hormone balance and healthy skin, but through peak times of change in our lives (i.e. puberty, pregnancy, menopause) these shifts in testosterone and your metabolism can make the skin more oily, causing acne.

And of course there are cycles within cycles, so acne at the same time each and every month also gives you clues as to what may be up with your hormones.

ACNE ON THE
TEMPLES MAY BE
RELATED TO THE
LIVER AND UNHAPPY
DETOXIFICATION.

ACNE AROUND THE
MOUTH AND FOREHEAD
IS MORE LIKELY
RELATED TO
GUT HEALTH.

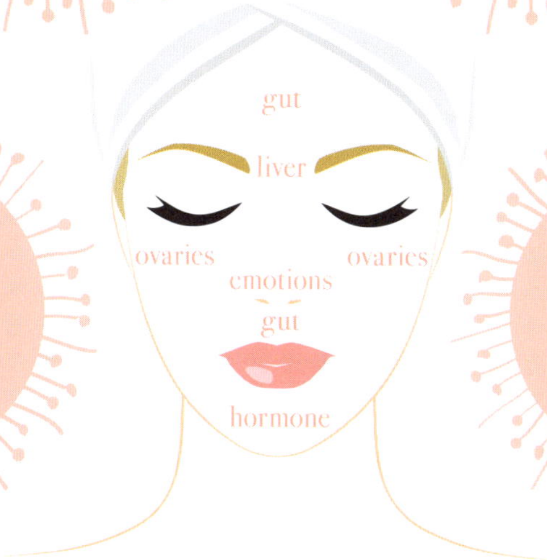

gut

liver

ovaries

emotions

ovaries

gut

ACNE ON THE
NOSE MAY BE
EMOTION RELATED.

ACNE ON THE
CHEEKS MAY BE
PCOS RELATED.

hormone

ACNE THAT APPEARS
ALONG THE JAWLINE
POINTS BACK TO
HORMONE IMBALANCE.

ACNE ON THE BACK
AND CHEST IS MORE
INDICATIVE OF ELEVATED
ANDROGENS LIKE
TESTOSTERONE.

ACNE ACCORDING TO THE MENSTRUAL CYCLE

DURING THE PERIOD

Because of higher testosterone, sebum glands are overactive, resulting in acne.

END OF THE PERIOD

From a TCM viewpoint, this would be due to blood deficiency. Nourishing the body with red and dark-coloured vegetables may be useful.

OVULATION

The peak in testosterone at this time encourages more oil production. Make sure you're loving your liver in this phase if you do see acne.

PRE-PERIOD

As progesterone builds, it causes the skin to swell and the pores are forced shut. This can lead to acne.

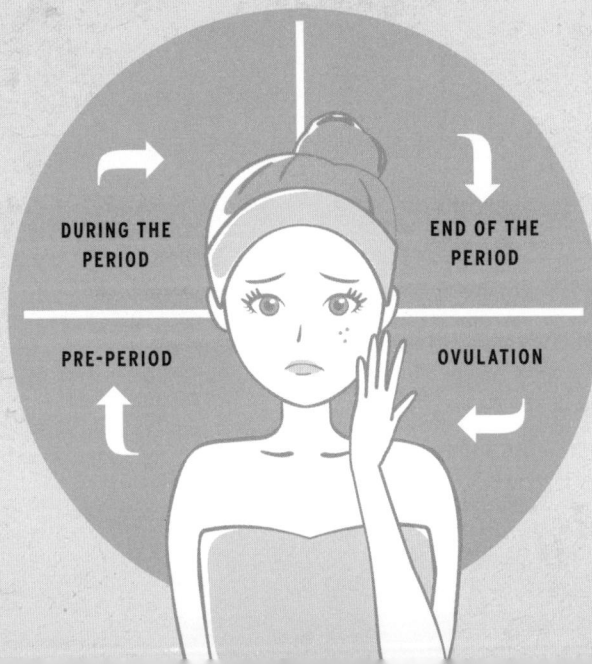

DURING THE PERIOD

END OF THE PERIOD

PRE-PERIOD

OVULATION

Women with PCOS may find they have very early onset acne as the adrenals may activate earlier. This also means there is a relationship between the severity of acne and stress, since your adrenals are the gland that sit on top of your kidneys and are responsible for the release of your main stress hormones, cortisol and adrenaline.

An increase of stress will increase the amount of stress hormones released into the body. This can lead to an increase in sebum production. But also, increased cortisol in the body leads to increased inflammation and, in a nutshell, acne is inflammation. Chronic stress will undoubtedly increase the severity of skin conditions such as acne, eczema, rosacea, vitiligo (when patches of skin become lighter) and urticaria (hives). **Skin changes aren't just limited to acne but may show up as rashes, lumps or bumps, too.**

When it comes to other skin irritations and other skin issues, nothing actually changes much in terms of treatment. Again, the gut is the first point of call and we must begin to nurture it to really treat any skin problems, so it's important that we first work from the inside out, otherwise we'll only ever end up treating the symptoms and not the long game. I have a few tips when it comes to addressing skin problems, especially acne.

TREATING ACNE

I. Combat inflammation

Many skin conditions are also a result of crazy inflammation due to poor diet. Inflammatory foods, including gluten, sugar and dairy, can wreak havoc with our insides and really wear away good gut flora. My suggestion is to apply the 80/20 rule (avoiding these inflammatory foods 80% of the time and letting your hair down the other 20%). You might like to pick one of these foods and remove it (say, soy or gluten) as a start and see where that takes you. Gluten is a disaster for most people, it's super hard to digest and leads to a sizeable amount of problems, all because of the inflammation it may cause. Cut it out for a few weeks as a starting point and see.

2. Cleanse

If your acne or poor skin is a result of toxic build up, it might be time to cleanse. (A cleanse can also really help acne due to hormone imbalance.) In a perfect world we wouldn't need to detoxify but sadly pollutants are everywhere; found in our water, air, food and environment in general. Let it be noted, cleanses don't need to be harsh and drastic. I run a very simple cleanse on my website, www.natkringoudis.com, that is all about eating really easily digested foods, cleaning out the gut and regulating the liver gently. It's a free 5-day program. A gentle reboot can be incredible for better hormone balance too. If this isn't your thing, simply start by increasing fibre and adding more water to your routine.

3. Rebalance your hormones

Of course that's why you're here, but when it comes to specifically treating your skin it can be the one thing you've been missing. Hormonal acne is most often seen along the jawline and commonly on the neck and back. If this is where you're finding your trouble spots to be (and often they are way worse than spots – they are boulders big enough to seal a tomb – I should know, I'm totally prone myself), it's your clue to getting onto rebalancing. Generally, I find that in these instances women are oestrogen dominant. Learn more about excess oestrogen in the following pages.

4. Know your triggers and avoid or manage

I know for me, lack of sleep, flying and that special little window before my pending period are all times that my skin can go a little haywire. So it's in these times I need to step it up with good nutrition and quality filtered water. Diet and lifestyle play a huge role in facilitating the nutrients our bodies need to nourish our skin – remember food will either help you keep your health in top form or it will bring it down to the ground. It's in these times we might need to nurture ourselves a little better and be mindful that putting our bodies under extra stress will only make the situation worse. My biggest fix is actually a nice cup of tea and a good night's sleep. While the type of tea can be therapeutic (my favourites to assist at this time are chamomile or licorice tea), this simple act of taking a load off is maybe just as beneficial as the tea itself.

5. Find your topical fix

It took me years to realise that my skincare regimen was actually part of the problem. I was madly trying to strip away the oil, which only made the issue worse. The more I tried to scrub and lather, the more my skin was being stripped of essential natural oils, meaning it was constantly being tripped into overdrive. The solution for me was oil cleansers combined with a good old face washer! I generally advocate this for my patients no matter what their skin type, since oil for me was my saviour, but equally we are all different, so it's important to work out what works best for your skin type. My best recommendation is to invest in some time with a natural skin care provider and really get to understanding individually what your skin needs.

SUPPLEMENTS FOR THE SKIN (AND HORMONE IMBALANCE IN GENERAL)

Fibre mix I like to combine psyllium, flaxseed (linseed), slippery elm and chia as a morning ritual to really keep hormones happy. Combine 2 parts each psyllium and slippery elm to 1 part each of flaxseed (linseed) and chia; keep the mix in an airtight jar and take 1 teaspoon each morning in diluted juice or water. This can be enough to sweep the digestive system, regulate the liver, move out any toxins as well as act as a prebiotic (those are the essentials to feed the good gut bacteria).

Fish oil Excellent for nourishing the skin, fish oil is full of amino acids and helps to look after your healthy glow. Remember - you get what you pay for, so make quality count. I prefer capsules over the oil itself as it is simpler to take and less offensive.

Zinc May be taken as a supplement but is also found in greens, pumpkin seeds and sesame seeds. Excellent to balance hormones and strengthen the gut integrity, meaning your digestive system is less likely to 'leak' and therefore helps to reduce inflammation.

Probiotics Fermented foods plus prebiotics and probiotics are the keys to healthy skin since the gut and the skin are so close in their relationship. Overgrowth of unhealthy bacteria will contribute to skin issues, especially influencing the microbes externally.

As with all supplements, consult with your qualified healthcare professional before taking.

Mood swings and PMS

Hormone changes aren't just physical, we feel them emotionally too, and mood swings are the ultimate example. Maybe you've experienced words flowing from your mouth that didn't feel like they belonged to you but you said them anyway, almost as if you had no control over yourself and they just splattered their way out like verbal diarrhea. Or maybe you've felt your emotions swing so fiercely from happy to rage you lived your very own re-enactment of beauty and the beast. Your sex hormones, especially oestrogen (testosterone can cause mood swings for boys), may be largely at play here, as they are responsible for rewiring emotional processing areas of the brain. With TCM we can add another layer to this and look at the specific emotions that may be most commonly experienced and we can help to even out the emotions a little more. Also, as we've learnt, emotions are there to be felt and serve a purpose; it's when we're down more than we are up that it might be time to recruit support.

Premenstrual Tension (PMT) or Premenstrual Syndrome (PMS) are the terms used to refer to a bucket load of symptoms that may occur anytime from ovulation onwards, during the luteal phase. More commonly, in the few days leading up to a period, we can feel heightened emotions. We may feel more sensitive or vulnerable alongside other common symptoms such as breast tenderness or tingly nipples, acne, headaches, lower back pain and period pain. Some women can experience these symptoms for up to two weeks before the period. While PMS is considered normal, it doesn't have to be there and is your body's own way to yet again let you know that something has to give. Stress is a very common cause of PMS.

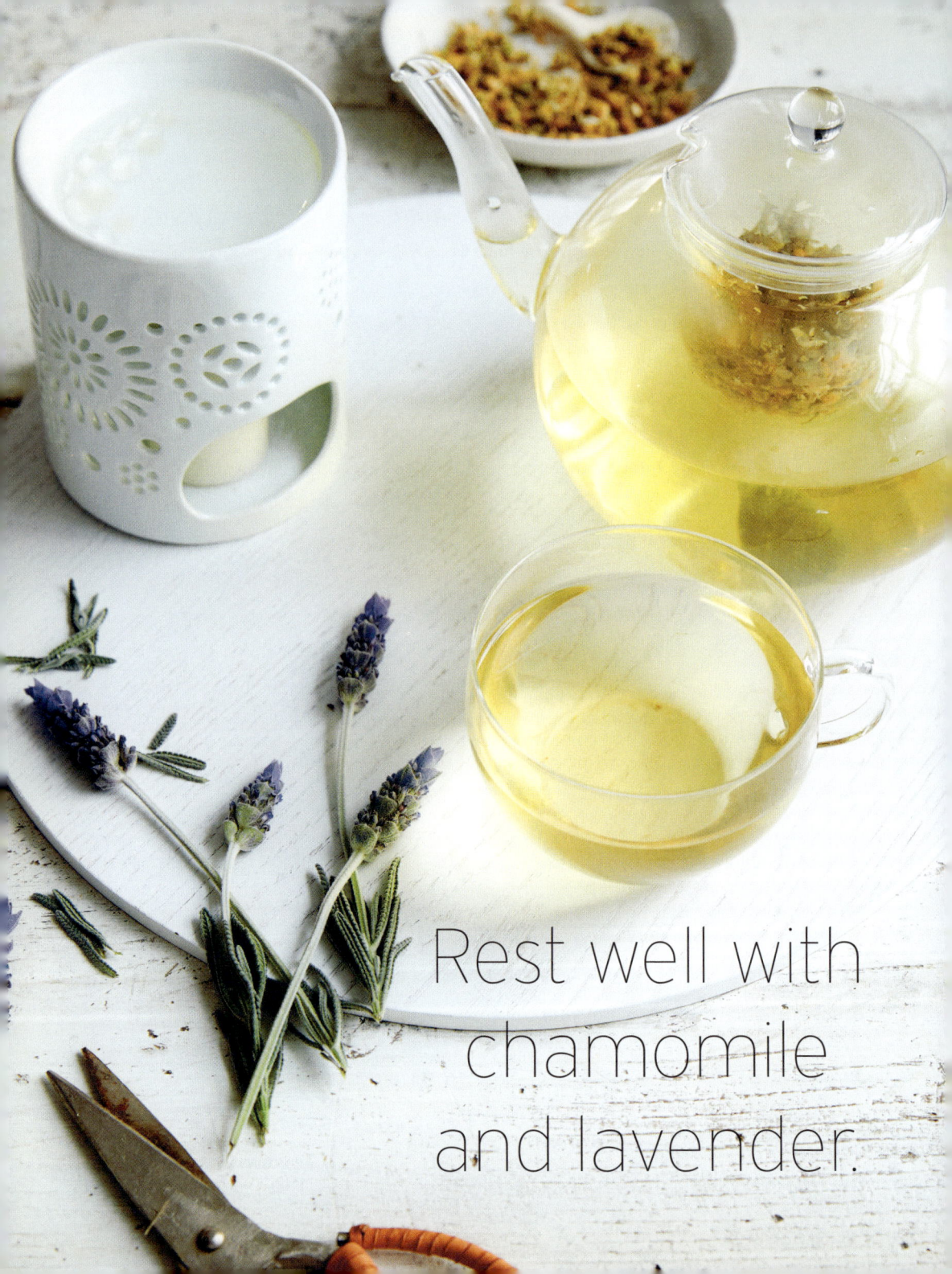

Rest well with chamomile and lavender.

I've listened to many patients (and friends) lamenting about their painful PMS symptoms, and the irrational desire to 'kill anyone who comes near me'. Now we all have a bit of a laugh, and pull out the chocolate and the hot water bottles, but there are some nasty side effects to deal with during menstruation. It can all seem a bit much and totally unfair. Here are some of my favourite fixes.

TACKLING PMS

1. Chamomile tea

(More tea! It truly is a wonderful fix.) It will help to keep you calm and can also help alleviate cramping associated with menstrual bleeding. It has also been found to be mildly sedating and therefore relaxes nerves. Nice one to have on standby!

2. Go easy

As we've discussed, in the premenstrual window, we are best to pull up and go gently. This may mean a night or two on the couch or cancelling a meeting or event. The rest time is essential. Do something nice for yourself – get a facial or a massage and really take advantage of some 'you' time.

3. Vitamin B

Load up on foods (or supplements) that contain B vitamins to immediately balance out oestrogen and boost the feel-good hormones, dopamine and serotonin. Foods rich in B's include eggs, meats, organic chicken and fish.

4. Gentle exercise

Choose exercise that is perfect to gently stretch out the body, improve circulation and ease tension. Get bendy – grab your yoga mat and stretch (a simple child's pose or a hip flexor stretch can really help). The movement can be wonderful to help increase blood flow and alleviate pain.

5. Rest

Menstruation is a big deal for your body and resting isn't being indulgent but necessary (after all, you are listening to your body more now, right?). You may feel extra tired for the first few days of your period – listen to the wisdom of your body, it is telling you this for a reason. Being in bed by 10 pm is essential – from a TCM perspective, this is when your body renews blood.

6. Lavender oil

It is an instant mood lifter and aids in easing tension. Plus it smells good! Add a few drops to a bath, on your pillow or use in a diffuser.

7. Sunshine

Get a little sunshine in. Without doubt sunshine lifts serotonin, our feel good hormone which not only regulates mood but also sleep, appetite and digestion. One sure way to put a smile on your dial is to spend just 5 minutes under the sun's rays.

Once you get past PMS and the onset of the period, you may feel a great sense of relief. Remember, it's best to just chill out for a few days while your body does what it needs to do. And while PMS, period pain and woes are considered 'normal', they don't have to be there. As we're learning, there's so much you can do to identify why you have these frustrating symptoms and find long-lasting solutions to fix the problem at its core.

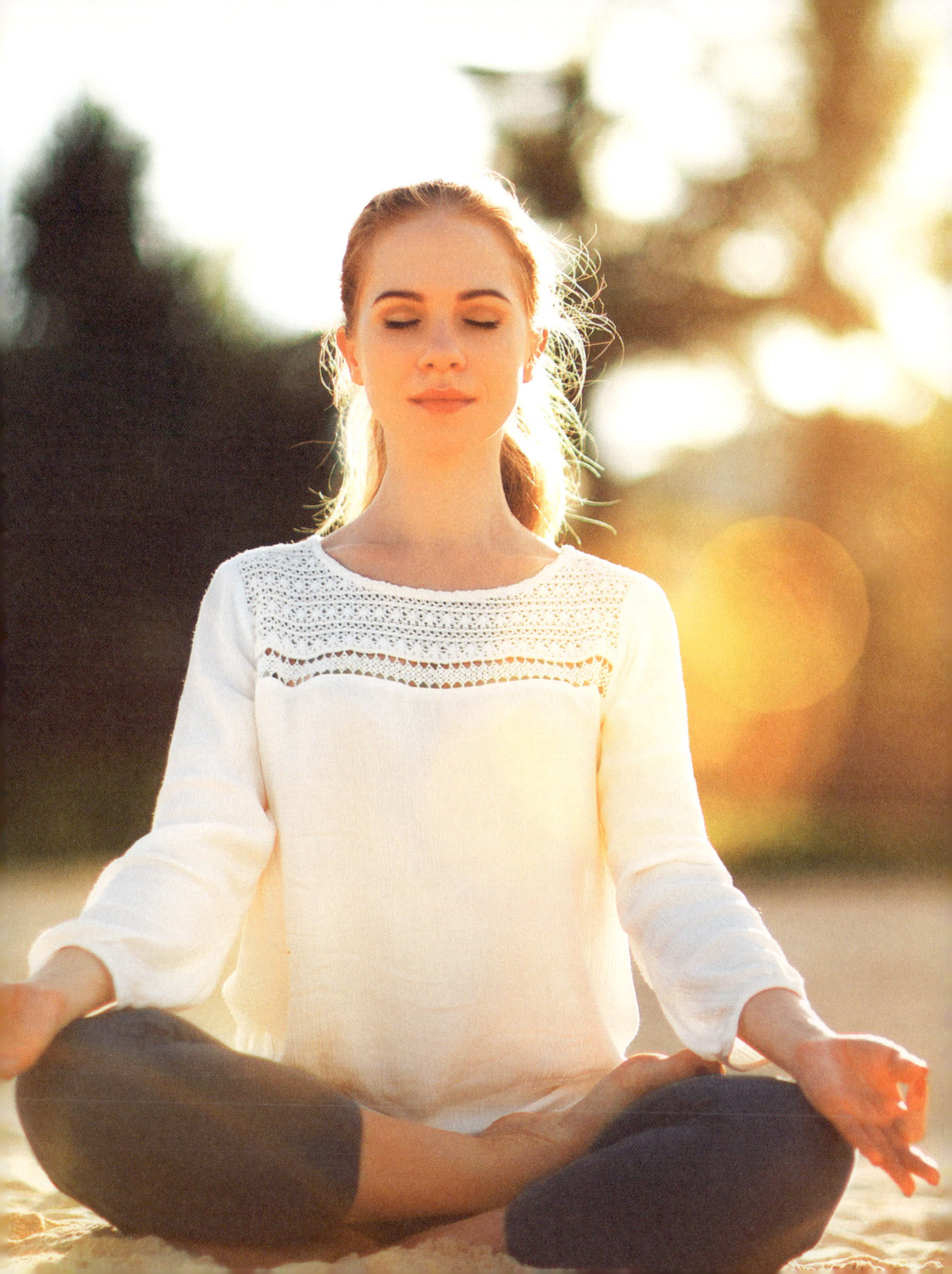

SUPPLEMENTS FOR MOOD SUPPORT

Magnesium Increase your dose leading into peak hormone times (pre-ovulation for around 3 days and the same premenstrually for around 3 days). I recommend seeking the best quality you can find at your health food store. You can take the recommended dose and in these peak times, add in an extra midday dose safely as your body requires more during this time.

B vitamins As already mentioned, these are great destressors and PMS fixers.

Maca Excellent for hormone imbalance and very safe to take. You can add this to smoothies as a powder or take in supplement form.

Consult with your doctor before taking supplements in case they may react with other medications.

WORKSHEET: **SWITCH IT UP**

Fill in this page when it's time to take charge of your emotions.
Write down the most dominant emotion.

_____

Why do you feel like this?

_____

Will it still be an issue in a week's time?

_____

Is there anything you can do now to make it better?

_____

What could help you to feel better now?

_____

Could you talk to somebody about it?

_____

Write down reflections and feelings after you've slept
on it or had some time out.

_____

Bloating

Bloating may be due to several factors and often we turn to our digestive system as the cause. This isn't incorrect and very often can be the reason why your stomach may feel like you've consumed a watermelon, rind and all. But your hormones may also be at play. How do you know if it's lunch or your luteal phase? The following image explains.

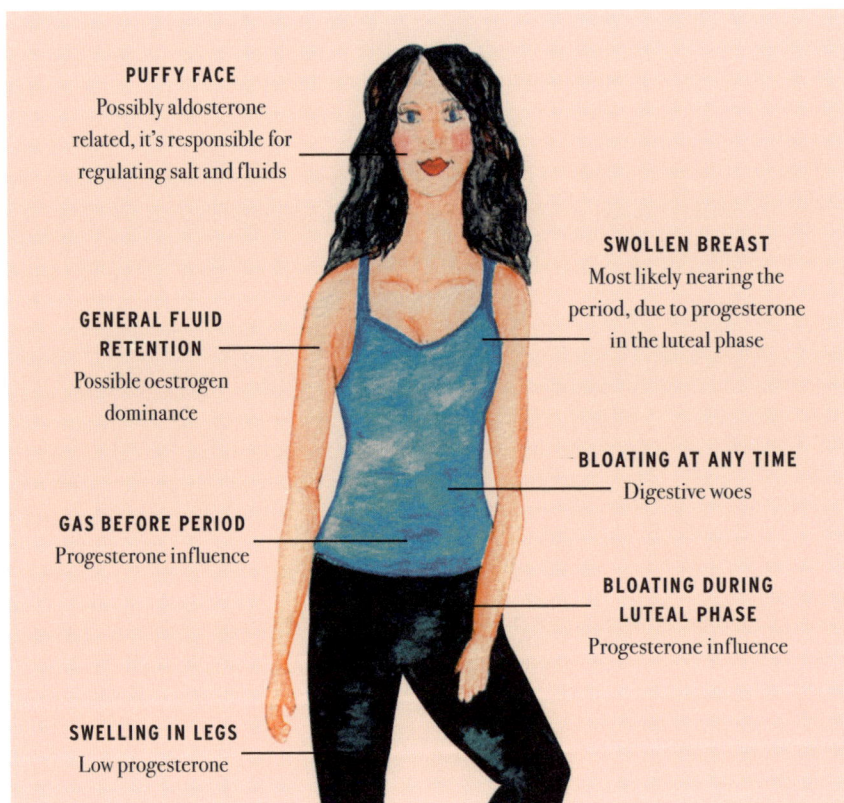

PUFFY FACE
Possibly aldosterone related, it's responsible for regulating salt and fluids

SWOLLEN BREAST
Most likely nearing the period, due to progesterone in the luteal phase

GENERAL FLUID RETENTION
Possible oestrogen dominance

BLOATING AT ANY TIME
Digestive woes

GAS BEFORE PERIOD
Progesterone influence

BLOATING DURING LUTEAL PHASE
Progesterone influence

SWELLING IN LEGS
Low progesterone

BEATING THE BLOAT

We are living at a time where our gut health is severely compromised. Hands down, the number one reason I see health issues in my clinic is because of this reason alone. It's simple. If we can't adequately assimilate and absorb nutrients from our food and drink, we find ourselves severely overfed and undernourished – we eat far more food than we need, to meet our body's nutritional requirements and even then, we are barely scraping in.

Bloating will begin to happen when our digestive system struggles to do its job. If it is out of kilter, one of the first symptoms to show up is bloating. This is only amplified by foods we find difficult to digest – the main offenders being gluten, dairy and sugar. Perhaps we are born with compromised gut health (we immediately inherit our mother's gut health at conception), or other factors during our lifetime like the pill, antibiotics or other medications have contributed. In any case, sub-average gut health can be one of the reasons we experience bloating. Overgrowth of certain (unwelcome) bacteria in the gut can also contribute to gas and bloating, should food build up in the digestive tract and not get moved through efficiently.

Other foods may also contribute to bloating. Beans and onions are high on the offender list but, depending on the state of your gut, other foods like grains may too be the culprit. I literally only have to look sideways at quinoa and I'm bloated for days. (Ok a fair stretch of the truth but seriously I find it way too difficult to digest.) For those with intolerances, this can also affect your digestive system. Eating fruit on a full stomach can lead to bloating too as it begins to ferment in the gut. Oh and don't forget, many raw and cold foods can be super hard to digest and cause the tummy to blow up like a balloon. Since your gut digests at around 37°C (98°F), it really has to go to work when food is raw and cold. For some, by the time it performs this task alone, it is near exhaustion and breaking down the food is a near impossible task.

But here's my absolute favourite. You get to blame your hormones once again (because who hasn't said – oh I'm so hormonal!?). Bloating can also be something we suffer from depending on where we are in our menstrual cycle. In the lead up to ovulation, we experience a final peak in oestrogen before it drops off to let progesterone do its thing. Along with this rise in oestrogen, we can see an increase in water retention, especially when oestrogen dominance is at play. The same can happen in the lead up to the period arriving, so depending on where you are in your cycle, you might want to track your bloating alongside this information to really get some answers.

> To see if bloating is triggered by hormonal fluctuations, keep a diary of when the bloating occurs and how that relates to your menstrual cycle.

There are a host of things that will contribute to the tummy billowing out to resemble a pregnant woman. It's not fun and, at best, it's uncomfortable. So how do you know if you are suffering from being bloated or if the issue is a more permanent fixture? **To put it simply – weight, especially around the tummy, doesn't quickly come and go like the effects of bloating.**

Bloating tends to come and go and if you can pinpoint your triggers, you can start to allow this to guide you as to what is going on inside your digestive system. It is typically only around the stomach and not anywhere else, although fluid retention can add to the confusion and we can hold fluid in various parts of our body. This too tends to come and go, unlike stubborn adipose tissue.

Bloating can last hours and sometimes days, depending on the trigger (typically gluten attacks can be long lived) and the state of the gut but if you are constantly eating foods that your body can't deal with, your bloating might seem like a more permanent fixture.

However, all of these factors that can cause bloating can also lead to weight gain. Sluggish digestion leads to overeating, hormone imbalance and is just another form of stress your body doesn't necessarily know how to handle. So what might begin as bloating can soon turn into something more long term, if not addressed.

Breast changes

Some of us have bigger 'chests' than others, some are still waiting for the day they will arrive (that's still me ... I don't think they are coming!) but whatever your caper, when those changes start happening they can be completely painful and totally weird. Breast buds generally begin forming around 9 or 10 years of age where small or hard lumps begin to be felt. Not only do they begin to become quite sore, they can often feel itchy or burning. While you may not physically see growth, you may certainly feel it. More annoying even, one can grow more rapidly than the other, leaving you feeling rather lopsided. Your nipples may also be sensitive and change. I recall that feeling, it was literally like muscle soreness times by 10!

It's really normal for breasts to start to grow anytime from 8 years of age, and can happen as late as 12. There's no real rush and the timing of the growth doesn't really mean much at all; it certainly doesn't impact the size that your breasts will grow to as that is determined by your genetics more than anything else. Most commonly, the breast buds will begin to develop approximately one year before the period arrives.

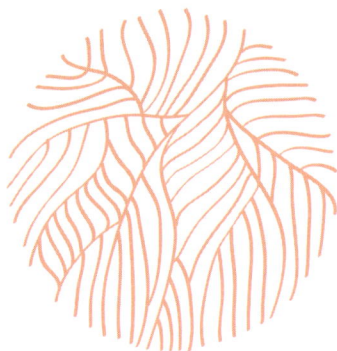

BREAST FORMATION

At 9-10 years of age the 'breast buds' form. They may feel like a little blueberry under each nipple. The breast bud is made up of the nipple, areola (which is the coloured skin around the nipple) and the lump underneath. You may also notice the colour of the nipples and areola begin to change.

- Breasts may be tender, burning, itchy and sensitive to materials over them.
- Breasts may also be lopsided – buds normally start on one side and then the other.
- Breasts may hurt when you run or walk.
- Breasts may be lumpy.
- Breasts may develop small pimple-like dots, which is no problem.

STAGES OF PUBERTY

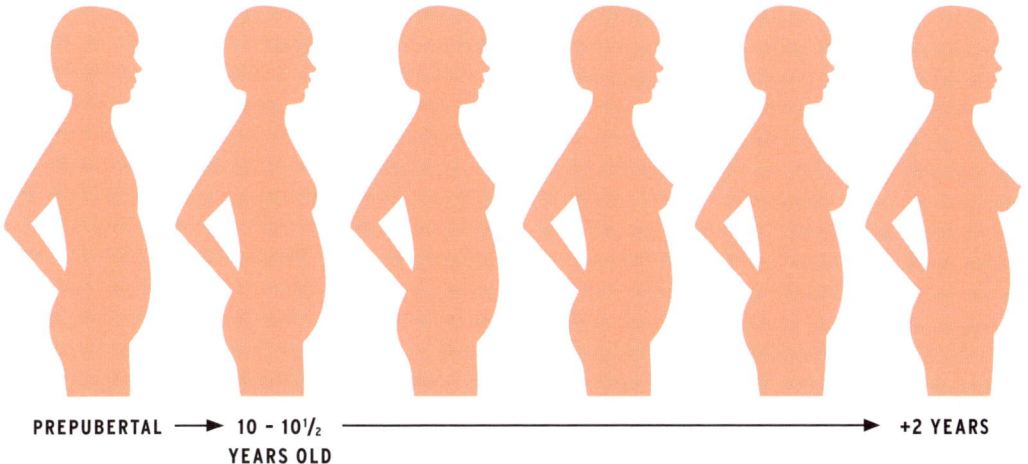

PREPUBERTAL → 10 - 10½ YEARS OLD ————————————→ +2 YEARS

Changes 'down there'

You may have freaked out the first time you saw discharge or mucus in your underpants or felt like you'd wet yourself the first few times your period arrived. All perfectly normal. As outlined, mucus is part of the healthy vagina flora and your best guide in knowing that your body is working properly since it can tell you so much information about what is going on 'in there'.

Pubic hair obviously makes its way onto your labia majora (the outer folds of skin surrounding the vagina) and slowly but surely sets in. This is not going to let up. But don't worry, we're all in the same boat. It's of course not limited to the pubic region but also appears in your armpits too. Just like the hair on your head, your pubic hair can be characteristically different to your best friend's. Some are short and curly and others are long and straight, and just because you're one or the other doesn't really matter. It doesn't mean anything specifically, nor does the amount you have matter. The most important part of it all is that it grows.

Perhaps you're wondering what's the point of pubic hair? It may seem rather unnecessary. I'm here to tell you it's not there to keep your nether regions warm in the unlikely event of a blizzard when your underpants are down but rather acts as a cushion to prevent friction and protect your most sensitive areas of your body from damage or injury. It also helps to protect from certain harmful bacteria or germs. Some prefer to remove it, be it partially or fully. While it is a matter of personal choice, as unwanted as it might be, it is there for a good reason.

Newsflash: your vagina may not ever smell like a bed of roses and at times when you've been out in the heat or perhaps skipped a shower it may have a slightly unpleasant odour. In normal circumstances, when you are taking good care of your most intimate body parts, they shouldn't smell bad (as we outlined previously) but, add the wrong material (synthetic is a common culprit) or a hot sweaty day to the mix and it can be the perfect combination for something that smells nothing short of the finest blue vein cheese your nose has ever come near. There are a few important guides you can follow to keep your vagina flora healthy and feeling fresh.

1. WASH REGULARLY.

Your everyday shower is important for overall good hygiene. You may feel a little more on the nose during period time and if you feel like the extra shower, please do yourself a favour, treat yourself to the kind gesture and take it. Avoid soaps and perfumes around your vagina, warm water and a washcloth is perfect – nothing more is needed.

2. KEEP YOUR UNDERPANTS ON CIRCULATION.

Changing your underwear each time you shower is perfect. If you feel like at certain times of the cycle you need to change them a little more often, do.

3. USE ESSENTIAL OILS.

These can be wonderful for all kinds of ailments. Tea tree oil is excellent as it is antimicrobial and a natural antibiotic. Dab only a drop or two (no more) onto a warm washcloth and gently sponge the area. If there is any bacterial overgrowth, this will assist.

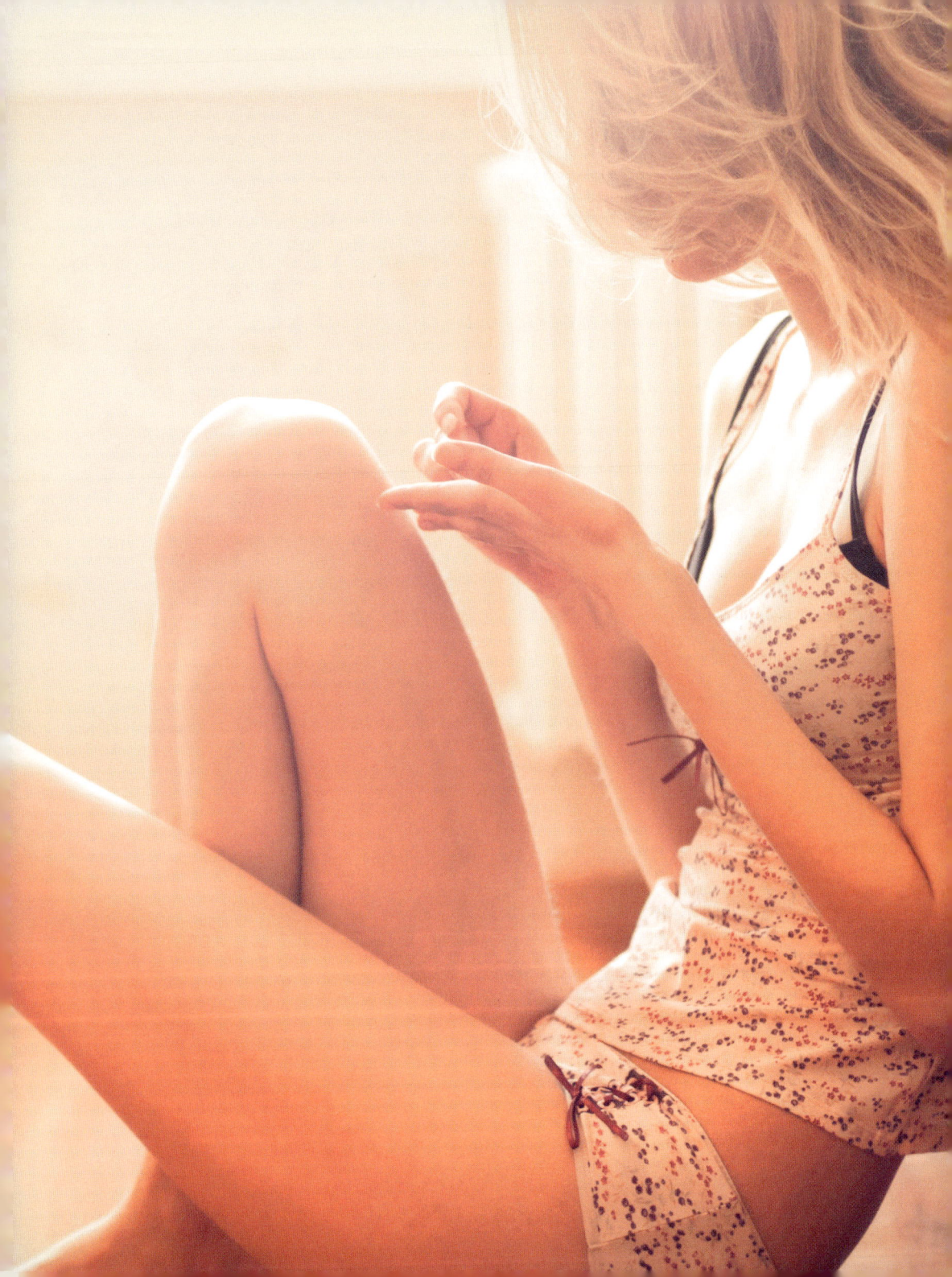

If you're still worried about the smell of your vagina, it may be useful to have it checked. Issues like thrush, Urinary Tract Infections (UTIs) or overgrowth of bacteria can be characterised by an odd smell and are often accompanied by other symptoms, such as increased discharge, burning sensations, and, in some instances, fever or other signs of infection. It's certainly not something to fear but best be checked out by your doctor in case a more appropriate treatment needs to be administered.

Should you find yourself in a situation where you continue to get recurrent infections like UTIs or thrush, it may be a sign that your flora needs a little care. Everything you're learning in this book is taking you one step closer towards better health overall and it is certainly a move in the right direction when you apply these principles. Gut health is without a doubt the best starting point here.

RECURRENT UTI TREATMENT

Commonly, I will see in the clinic women who encounter recurrent UTIs at the same time of their cycle, most often during their period and sometimes at ovulation. This may be due to the characteristic changes caused by hormones during these active times of the cycle. Progesterone also is believed to have an influence on the gut, which is another factor thought to contribute.

A WORD ON ANTIBIOTICS

Often antibiotics are prescribed for recurrent infections (of course not limited to UTIs but for infections in general), which may assist in treatment of bacterial infections. It is important to note when using the marvels of antibiotics for any health condition that you support the body at the same time. Unfortunately, not only do antibiotics go to war with the unwanted bacterial overgrowth, they also may have their way with your precious good bacteria too, leaving your body vulnerable, which may be one of the reasons your infection keeps on making a comeback – your body simply has no fight left to give. What's more, the world of understanding your microbiome is coming along faster than the next lunar eclipse and blue moon combination, and we're beginning to learn so much more about this area of health.

Stay tuned and keep your ear to the ground with this, it's a very important part of your health that can't be dismissed. If you choose to or need to take antibiotics for your infection, here's what to do:

- If you do nothing, nothing changes. Antibiotics aren't a magic bullet, it's all of the other little things that you do while you're taking them that counts most. These can be adopted as a treatment alongside antibiotics but also can be used as a stand-alone treatment. Of course if UTIs persist, consult your healthcare professional.

- Avoid inflammatory foods while taking antibiotics – these include gluten, sugar and dairy. These foods impact the digestive system and cause your cells to work harder (and not smarter). Leave them off the list if you can while taking an antibiotic course.

- Add in fermented foods or prebiotics and probiotics, which help to support and promote healthy bacteria. Prebiotics are common in everyday foods like asparagus or slippery elm. These foods help feed the good bacteria. I've included lists in Chapter 4. Probiotic foods contain live bacteria that are supportive of healthy body function, essential to life itself. The trick is – don't overdo it, you'll feel awful as you experience 'die off' when the good bacteria battle it out with the not so good.

Slowly and surely is the key (start with approximately 1/2 a teaspoon per day of fermented foods to begin with and then increase slowly).

- When fighting infection it is imperative to drink plenty of water to assist in flushing the body, especially for thrush or UTIs. Approximately two litres per day is good.

- Include foods that naturally support good health. Manuka honey is a wonderful internal support. Garlic with its natural anti-inflammatory properties and immune-boosting goodness is great for treating infections. Slip it into your food at the first sign of an infection.

Herbs to treat UTIs

Occasional vaginal itching is also something that is common and usually nothing to worry about, although if it gets worse or is pesky it's worth having it checked by your doctor. Here are a few herbal fixes.

- **Dandelion:** Traditional Chinese Medicine calls on the benefits of Dandelion or Pu Gong Yin to assist in addressing painful urination. It helps to clear heat and inflammation and also to treat pain. You can use dandelion tea as a simple support.
- **Job's tears:** Known in Traditional Chinese Medicine as Yi Yi Ren, it also assists in strengthening the gut, clearing infection via urination and treating pain.
- **Cinnamon bark:** Aids in warming the body to 'unblock' and treat pain associated with UTIs. We frequently use cinnamon in TCM for pain. It offers great relief.

PCOS

As we mentioned, weight gain may be one of the early signs of Polycystic Ovarian Syndrome (PCOS) but it is not the only one. PCOS is a state of hormone imbalance where there are multiple 'cysts' (more correctly, follicles) on the ovaries resulting from excess androgens in the body (like testosterone – remember we need a little, just not enough for the entire football team). This is amplified with issues in insulin regulation and often inflammation. We are now at the point of understanding a lot more in the world of PCOS. We've recently uncovered that there are different types of PCOS, which has done wonders for its treatment – because nothing is one-size-fits-all and your symptoms may be wide and varied; however, these symptoms do generally remain at the crux of the issue and that's exactly where we must focus treatment for long-term health.

> It is estimated that approximately 20% of women of reproductive age have PCOS.

Typical symptoms of PCOS due to the presence of these excess androgens include missing or irregular periods, weight gain, acne, facial hair, thinning hair on the head and pelvic pain being the most common. However, in this fresh approach to PCOS, women who are lean or acne-free or even post-pill are also being diagnosed with multiple cysts and elevated androgens.

The Rotterdam criteria (named after the city of the study) is the testing method doctors use to diagnose PCOS. The three criteria in establishing this conclusion include:

I. Delayed ovulation or menstrual cycles (known as anovulation, meaning less than 10 menstrual cycles per year or cycles longer than 35 days).

2. Hyperandrogenism/high androgenic hormones like testosterone (confirmed via blood test).
3. Polycystic ovaries on ultrasound (12 or more present on each ovary).

To confirm PCOS, patients only need to present with two out of the three criteria. But because the world is constantly evolving (thank goodness!) and because we're defining that there are different forms or phenotypes of PCOS, patients don't necessarily present with the whole caboodle of symptoms.

Women with PCOS don't necessarily have acne or weight gain.

It's suggested that this testing will continue to evolve and, as research and time goes on, we will continue to understand more about PCOS and its triggers.

It's because of the tricky hormone imbalance that women are often told PCOS will impact their ability to have children and, left untreated, this is certainly a factor in 'infertility'. However, managed properly and from the get-go, PCOS can be controlled and for most is a treatable condition. Many women who have adopted the right diet, lifestyle and environmental influences have gone on to have many babies and live without symptoms. Thankfully, everything we outline in this book is perfect for hormone imbalance in terms of the diet and lifestyle you should be living, especially when there is a known hormone issue. For my patients with PCOS, it's important for them to track their cycles, no matter the length.

Use the diary in the back of this book to learn about your signs and symptoms and help you understand your body better. It will become your best friend.

In Chapter 1 we shared what a 'normal' period should look like. For women with PCOS, this may look slightly (or completely) different. Women with PCOS may still experience regular cycles, especially if they implement the right approach. For those who find their cycles are irregular, there are several reasons why.

POLYCYSTIC OVARIAN SYNDROME (PCOS) CHART

DAY	INFORMATION	DAY	INFORMATION	DAY	INFORMATION
1	Period	21	Moist	41	Dry
2	Period	22	Moist	42	Dry
3	Period	23	Moist	43	Dry
4	Period	24	Moist	44	Dry
5	Spotting	25	Wet	45	Dry
6	Dry	26	Wet	46	Dry
7	Dry	27	Dry	47	Dry
8	Moist	28	Dry	48	Dry
9	Moist	29	Dry	49	Dry
10	Dry	30	Dry	50	Dry
11	Dry	31	Dry	51	Dry
12	Dry	32	Dry	52	Dry
13	Moist	33	Dry	53	Dry
14	Moist	34	Dry	54	Dry
15	Moist	35	Dry	55	Dry
16	Dry	36	Dry	56	Dry
17	Dry	37	Dry	57	Dry
18	Dry	38	Dry	58	Period
19	Dry	39	Moist	59	
20	Dry	40	Wet	60	

*This is a sample chart. Your cycle might be different.

Women with PCOS may continue to attempt to ovulate over and over again. This is marked again, just like the cycle we spoke of earlier, by changes in cervical fluid patterns. I've also come to note in clinic that women with PCOS tend to have more cervical fluid in general, which can make it tricky to pinpoint when the body is attempting to ovulate. The trick for women with PCOS is to understand their body patterns and cervical mucus rhythm.

It's not impossible to discover your own rhythms, even when you have PCOS. Many women have regular cycles (albeit commonly longer) when experiencing PCOS; the important thing is to discover when you are ovulating. If you are getting a period, as we discussed in Chapter 1, you are more than likely ovulating.

PCOS doesn't make you infertile. The issue for women with PCOS is that while they have an oversupply of follicles, these eggs may or may not be able to be fertilised for conception.

Endometriosis

My period arrived without too much fuss. Sure, it looked murky and disgusting and nothing like I expected but there were no real issues. I didn't have period pain as a young teenager, nor did I feel like I got crazy hormone fluctuations, although my mother may tell you a very different story on the mood front. I grew up in a house where there were wholefoods on tap 24/7. My mother was quite invested in natural health care, prompted mostly by the death of her mother from terrible health when my mother was just 30 years of age. It's fair to say it hit home hard and motivated her to care for her own health and of course our health as a family on an entirely new level. Personally, as a kid growing up with this kind of lifestyle, I hated it. I resented the food in my lunch box (yes, Mum made my lunch until I was 18 years old, something I took for granted!!) and used to swap out my beautiful lunch for whoever was willing to trade their white bread and peanut butter sandwiches.

During my later years in high school, as with all teens, the pressure was on to perform, do my best and manage my social life (the latter probably being the highest priority – even though now I know better). It wasn't until stress really built for me as a young woman that my cycles began to become troublesome, possibly coupled by my new-found love for earning money and no longer having to necessarily tuck into my mum's wholesome cooking. I started to gain weight and experience really painful periods. I became that girl who would pass out from the pain some months, experience debilitating nausea and vomiting, and I would often find myself lying on the bathroom floor with my face pressed up against the tiles trying my best to get some relief, not only from period pain but also from the sensation that my face was burning up. My skin was a mess and my stomach seemed constantly bloated.

I moved away from home when I was just 18 years of age to begin life in the big smoke and to study. As I began to fend for myself, prepare my own meals, burn the candle at both ends and live the life of a uni student, my symptoms didn't improve; in fact they got worse – much worse. I endured many years of excruciating pain and suffering each menstrual cycle and also began to notice mid-cycle pain each month. My local KFC was my favourite haunt (it was literally 2 minutes up the road) and late nights were a common occurrence. I made no connection whatsoever to my lifestyle and my health. It never occurred to me that the life I was living was impacting my physical symptoms outside of feeling tired or having dry skin. But it does. And it was.

During this time, my weight continued to climb and I found myself feeling completely unwell. Not motivated by my nasty periods but by how unhappy I was with how I felt in my skin, I signed up to the gym and began to shift my diet more towards what I had been taught as a child. I quit KFC, started drinking more water and began investing in myself. It felt good to feel healthy and, within several weeks, I noticed I felt less bloated, my pants were feeling comfortable again and on the whole I had more energy and improved wellbeing. So I kept at it. I still hadn't made the connection between my happier menstrual cycles and my altered lifestyle but in hindsight it was no mistake that everything improved. Even my eczema went away – it's not something I've seen for more than 15 years. Life just got better all round.

While I was never formally diagnosed with endometriosis, knowing what I know now, it's fair to say all the signs were there. I wish I knew then what I know now and how simple changes in my day-to-day world would have made the biggest difference. Still to this day, if I have a stressful month I may experience some pain. On a scale of 1 to 10 (something I invite you to chart if you experience pain), it would be a 2 nowadays, compared to an 8 or 9 in those teen years and early 20s.

Endometriosis occurs when cells that belong in the uterus make their way into other areas of the body uninvited – typically outside (but near) the uterus – and grow. (The most common site for endometriosis to hide is on the ovaries, causing painful cysts.) As endometriosis worsens, however, it can spread as far as the nose (cue nosebleeds at the period time – another sweet little sign our bodies show us when things go awry). Each month when we menstruate, our uterine lining should easily make its way out through the cervix and vagina. For women with endometriosis, those same cells that allow us to bleed every month may have migrated outside of the uterine cavity and want to do the same, the only difference being they don't necessarily have an easy escape route (like the vagina) for the blood and as a result terrible pain and cramping is common. This can, over time, lead to scarring, which is linked to fertility issues.

Endometriosis may be incredibly stubborn and most commonly doctors will suggest a laparoscopy as the best option on offer to diagnose and remove the endometrial tissue – a procedure that may offer you some relief. However, if you're only removing evidence of the problem (as part of the laparoscopy your gynecologist removes any endometriosis found), are we really fixing the problem? If we continue with our day-to-day action plan without change post surgery, endometriosis will most likely return. The age-old saying, 'do nothing, nothing changes', aptly applies but that said, many women manage their endometriosis by frequent surgeries as well as the most common of the synthetic hormones, be it in the Oral Contraceptive Pill (OCP) or the mirena (IUD: a small, T-shaped intrauterine device). If this worked, I wouldn't be here writing about it in detail. The fact around any imbalance in the body is that it is being driven by something in your world – your environment, your day-to-day habits, your stress levels, your diet, your environment and your mind. It can be super tricky to work out where to best make inroads into better health, so lucky for you that's where I come in.

Do nothing, nothing changes.

So there's hope. In fact, we must act and of course we can make our own way towards finding a true solution for these conditions – my hope for you is that it is without surgery or medications that typically come with a bucket-full of side effects. I'm not advocating that you don't see your doctor for endometriosis, too, but starting at surgery (for most) and working back from there personally seems a little shot gun-esque. But even if this is your choice, you don't need to wait to start on your path towards better health.

It all begins with the small lifestyle changes you can make each and every day. Beautifully, the same diet and lifestyle I advocate for is appropriate for all kinds of hormone issues that I believe all women, endometriosis or not, should follow. Ultimately, it's all about happy hormones and, since endometriosis is worsened by too much oestrogen and the influence of oestrogen-mimicking substances (such as alcohol, plastics, environmental pollutants, self-care products, poor water quality and other toxins found in our foods) as well as stress, we must get savvy around our choices to pave our own way towards better hormone health. If you don't step up to the plate and create change, nobody else will do it for you.

Ultimately, your wellbeing lies with just you.

Points to remember

Ask yourself – why is this happening to me? I can assure you, it's not because you're being punished, even though it may feel like it.

Who's advocating to treat the root cause rather than symptoms? Should you continue with the same diet and lifestyle, you can't expect miracles.

There are some pretty simple changes that must be made to overcome endometriosis, all of which we are getting to the bottom of here, together.

MY 'TACKLE ENDOMETRIOSIS' TIPS

1. Here we go again - get onto the gut (you see, it truly is the epicentre).

2. Regulate the liver for better oestrogen metabolism (start with the fibre mix I mentioned in the Acne section).

3. Reduce stress. Stress is at the core of all hormone issues. For ways to internally reduce stress, see Chapter 3.

4. Check in on emotional health. Emotions seem to be a common theme for women suffering from endometriosis.

5. Eat for health. Your recipes are coming up - this is a fabulous start.

ENDOMETRIOSIS FLOW CHART

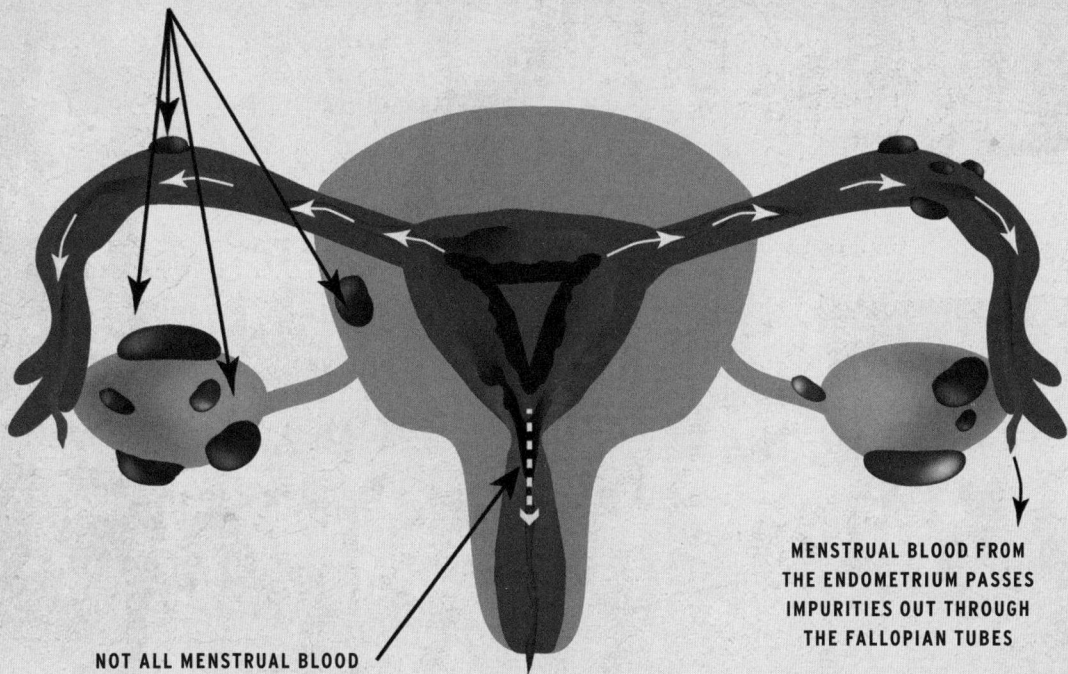

PIECES OF THE ENDOMETRIUM
TAKE ROOT. THESE ARE THE
LOCATIONS OF ENDOMETRIOSIS

MENSTRUAL BLOOD FROM
THE ENDOMETRIUM PASSES
IMPURITIES OUT THROUGH
THE FALLOPIAN TUBES

NOT ALL MENSTRUAL BLOOD
PASSES THROUGH THE VAGINA

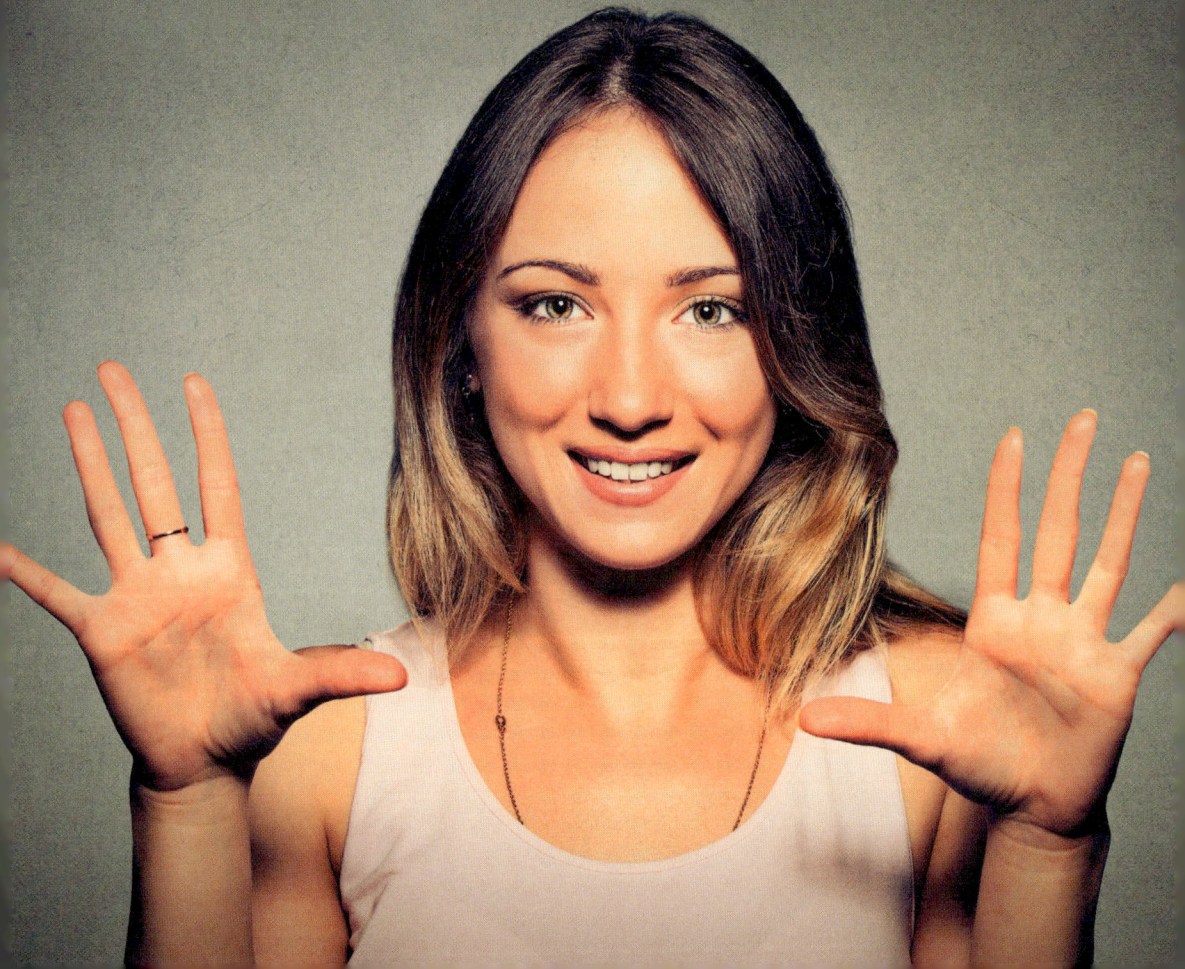

You are not alone.
Endometriosis
affects an estimated
1 in 10 women.

ADENOMYOSIS

A painful cousin to endometriosis is something called adenomyosis. Remember how endometriosis is when the lining of the uterus gets outside the tubes and sticks to places like the ovaries? Well, adenomyosis is when the lining, instead of staying confined to the inside of the uterus, grows roots and dives deep into the muscle. Think of it this way: imagine you're in the direct line of a cricket bat to the abdomen, every day for five days in a row. You could imagine that would hurt like the dickens and this is what your uterus feels like if you have adenomyosis. Now imagine if this happened every month for years. Over time, that poor uterus would just be sore all the time, but when you had the period it would hurt so much more. Another thing with this issue is that, because there is so much more lining, there is more surface area so these women have heavier, more painful periods. Doctors have a hard time diagnosing endometriosis and adenomyosis so they tend to want to put you on birth control pills as a fix, but it's important to recall that this may be a band-aid that isn't treating the root cause of the problem. This is fine for short-term relief but as a long-term solution it may not serve you well (because symptoms often break through birth control).

Painful periods

Pain at the period time is considered something many women experience and therefore 'the norm'. But I'm here to say, period pain isn't normal – and following on from endometriosis, just because you have period pain doesn't mean you have endometriosis either. I'd encourage you to grade your pain – the closer it is to 10, the quicker you need to listen to your body as it's a sure sign of inflammation and yet again, your body's own completely unfair way of telling you something is up. In almost all instances, it is treatable. If you are experiencing period pain, chances are there's probably a host of other symptoms that come with it, but once we start to address the true issues, many of these pesky sidekick symptoms clear up. Your symptoms are also more than likely to be different from those of your neighbour, her sister and their cousin and her bikini-waxer, because we are all different (yup, genetics!).

And remember, if you are using the pill as a means to treat period pain, you might like to understand that it isn't actually fixing the underlying causes – it's just masking the problem. It may serve some short-term relief for sure, but I'd always encourage you to look into the root of the issue rather than manage your symptoms alone.

During your period, your uterus is contracting to assist in the shedding of your uterine lining. Prostaglandins (hormone-like lipids made at the site of all injuries or, in this case, your menstrual bleeding) trigger these contractions in the uterus. Higher levels of prostaglandins are associated with more painful cramps; some women say high enough levels of prostaglandins can feel like labour. (Yes, doctors induce labour using prostaglandins.) But know that prostaglandins aren't exclusive to the uterus, in fact they are found in all tissues in the body. They are important in dealing with damage or infection that we may experience due to being injured or sick. They also control other natural processes, including blood flow, blood clots, the induction of labour during birth and inflammation. When there are more, there is evidently more pain – quite logically this tells us that addressing inflammation may assist with managing your pain better. Also, large amounts of prostaglandins released by the uterine lining can also make you feel feverish, nauseous, and overall flu-like.

When it comes to period pain, treating it isn't too different to endometriosis and the following quick fixes may be applied to both camps (endo or plain ol' period pain).

QUICK FIXES

Avoid cold foods at the period time

Eating cold and raw foods can be a huge contributor to menstrual cramping and pain. TCM suggests that pain is usually (in most instances) a result of blood or energy and nutrients not flowing freely; that is, there is either a blockage or something (for example, tissue scarring) in the way of the flow. You might have heard the term 'cold in the uterus' (everybody loves this one – it's a commonly diagnosed TCM condition). Women that present this way will most often experience quite substantial period pain that responds well to warmth and sometimes pressure, darker clotted blood flow and a cold body, especially in the lower abdomen at the period time. Switching to cooked foods at this time can be a great way to help keep symptoms under control – but remember, if it is bad, it might be time to seek a proper diagnosis.

Get the blood flowing – go for a walk

You need to be gentle at the period time – but this doesn't mean you can't exercise. Exercise can be wonderful to help treat period pain as it helps blood to flow through the reproductive organs. People who are what TCM diagnose as 'blood deficient' (meaning that they don't have adequate blood stores) may benefit most from this. These people are more likely to complain of draggy or dull pain at the period time, they can be dizzy or faint, cold and look pale. They may also find their menstrual blood looks pale and diluted.

Ease pain with tea (again!)

The heat from the tea will help increase blood flow and alleviate pain, but more than that, there are many teas that can be wonderful at this time. Chamomile is mildly sedative and therefore is useful to help treat pain. Raspberry leaf tea can also be useful to relax the uterus. Making a brew with ginger can also be useful to treat period pain. Studies show that it does so as it lowers pain-causing prostaglandins.

Sleep more

Plan extra sleep around the period time – when we are tired, we are more sensitive to everything. By getting adequate rest, the body is much happier for it – and if there are some period niggles, you cope much better when you are well rested. For me, 8 hours of sleep a night is a general rule and it's extremely important to be in bed by 10 pm so your body can rejuvenate well. TCM suggests that blood is built when we rest (and physiology suggests that sleep does more than just help us repair our body, it helps us detoxify and regenerate our hormones, too).

Eat for relief

Sound odd? Some foods will make pain better and others worse. Generally, wholefoods are always going to make your body happy. (I learnt the hard way!)

Exercise can help period pain.

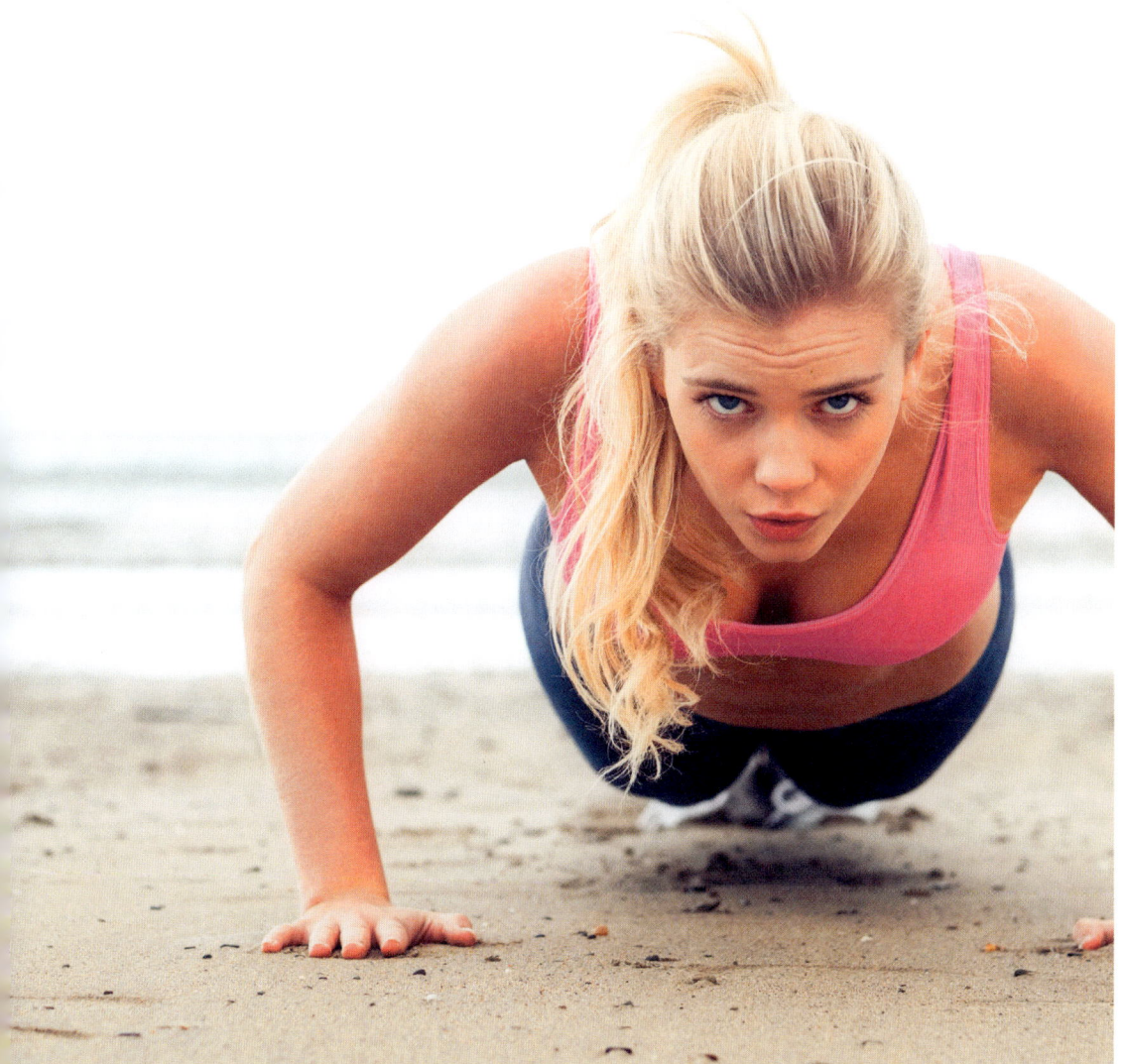

Foods that are high in fibre and good fats keep the bowels happy (if the bowel is strained, the pain can be worse) and the blood flowing, helping to ease pain. The top few include:

- Salmon or other oily fish
- Olive oil
- Nuts and seeds (soaked is best)
- Green leafy vegetables
- Aromatic spices – think turmeric, ginger, ground mustard, pepper.

If pain is really bad, it might be time to explore your options and find a solution that works for you. Remember to be kind to your body in the menstrual window, slowly and gently is the key. We love to push through and fight against it, but try as we might, this is never a good idea.

Be kind to your body; slowly and gently is the key.

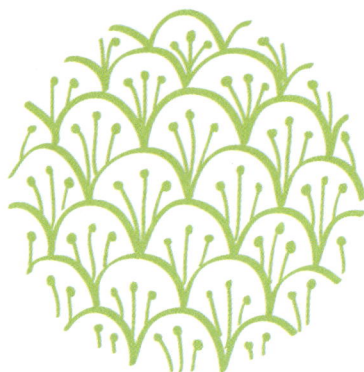

Missing periods

Your period is missing! Where and why did it go? When will it come back? Why is this bothering you so much when you've wished countless times for your period to go away anyways?

Anyone who has experienced amenorrhea knows about the anxiety caused by our friend who usually visits every month suddenly going M.I.A. I mean, how dare she just dip out on you when she's accompanied you (without invitation!) to so many dances, dates, beach weekends, and final exams?

Amenorrhea isn't a disease, curse, or illness, but rather a symptom of something else going on with your body (isn't everything?). Finding out exactly what is behind your amenorrhea can be tricky because it can be an indicator of many different issues.

The following are some of the main causes of amenorrhea.

MAIN CAUSES OF MISSING PERIODS

Hormone imbalances

For the most part hormonal imbalances are behind the majority of amenorrhea cases. Typically, the hormonal imbalance associated with amenorrhea is low oestrogen or a combination of low oestrogen and low progesterone.

When a woman's oestrogen and/or progesterone are too low, her body is unable to build up the uterine lining and subsequently shed that uterine lining each month (aka your period).

What exactly is causing this kind of hormonal imbalance can be one or a number of things. These are some of the top contributors:

- Hormonal birth control (especially the pill)
- Quitting hormonal birth control (post-pill amenorrhea)
- Eating disorders like anorexia or bulimia
- Exercising too much (gymnastics 7 times a week is definitely too much)
- Mental and emotional stress (including childhood abuse, be it emotional or physical)
- Low body weight
- Low thyroid function (hypothyroid)

Additionally, we can see the issue where we're producing too much testosterone. As you now know, high testosterone can actually prevent or significantly delay ovulation each month, which causes periods to become irregular or disappear completely. You guessed it, this problem is commonly diagnosed as Polycystic Ovarian Syndrome (PCOS).

Structural and genetic issues

These issues usually require more than just food and lifestyle changes. If you have any of these problems or conditions, chances are that you already know it. For instance, if you are experiencing primary amenorrhea, which means you've never had a period and you are 16 years or older, then one of these might apply to you and you should see a doctor to determine the cause.

- Asherman's syndrome – uterine scarring or adhesions, which can prevent blood from exiting the uterus.

- Pituitary tumour – which causes high levels of the hormone prolactin. Prolactin suppresses ovulation and menstruation.
- Mayer-Rokitansky-Küster-Hauser syndrome – underdeveloped reproductive organs or a lack of them.
- Other genetic structural abnormalities.

WHEN SHOULD I PANIC?

If the period hasn't arrived by the age of 15 (many doctors say 16 but I think being proactive is best), it may be time to run some tests. It's not necessarily anything to worry about - there's always a reason and addressing the root cause of this from a young age will mean your chances of having healthy hormones in years to come is far higher.

Medications

You know all those scary side effects that most medications list? Well, sometimes those lists include missing your monthly cycle. Discuss side effects with your doctor if you have questions or are feeling worried. Here are some meds that commonly cause amenorrhea:

- Hormonal birth control
- Antidepressants
- Blood pressure medicines
- Chemotherapy
- Allergy medications
- Antipsychotics

Natural reasons

Our body progresses through natural phases and cycles where sometimes amenorrhea is completely expected, so no need for alarm bells! These include:

- Rapid weight loss or weight gain
- Heightened stress over a period of more than one week
- Short and long distance travel

And of course the most obvious:

- Pregnancy
- Breastfeeding
- Perimenopause and menopause

Many women tell me that not having a period is a blessing or they don't want kids so why should they care about whether they have a period or not, but you should always seek adequate advice regarding missing periods. **Regardless of whether you want children or not, it is imperative to understand that your period health is reflective of your overall health. If your period is missing or irregular, something deeper is going on that you need to look at.**

Other symptoms

There are also many physical and emotional symptoms associated with amenorrhea that are no fun. These include:

- More acne than you've ever experienced in your life!
- Hair loss on your head or hair growth on your face (oh, the injustice of it all).

- Your sexy underwear stays in your drawer thanks to a low libido.
- Or worse ... when you do have sex, it hurts like hell.
- Low or no fertile cervical fluid – yes, sometimes your underwear can be too clean.
- Your energy is so low you can't get out of bed easily or even get through the day without caffeine or sugar.
- Depression or mood swings that disrupt your relationships and your life.

If you have not had a period for more than three months and you are experiencing any of the symptoms above, I highly recommend it's time to make some changes and, failing that, investigate further. The changes I advocate for in this book I'd recommend implementing for a period of 12 weeks and then reassessing your situation.

Why do these conditions develop?

As we discussed before, as with all conditions, we are genetically predisposed. This isn't something we can necessarily change; however, as we've discussed, it's all about outsmarting our genes and changing the variables that surround us to show our bodies how it's done. Your diet, lifestyle, environment and emotions are very powerful indeed!

Things change – it's a given. The trick with all things in life is to go with it, rather than against it. Nature teaches us this lesson every day.

CHAPTER 5

Your body challenges

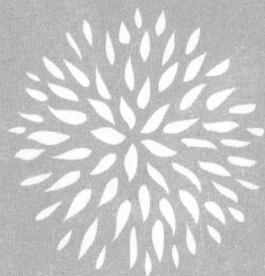

'Some changes look negative on the surface but you will soon realise that space is being created in your life for something new to emerge.'

ECKHART TOLLE

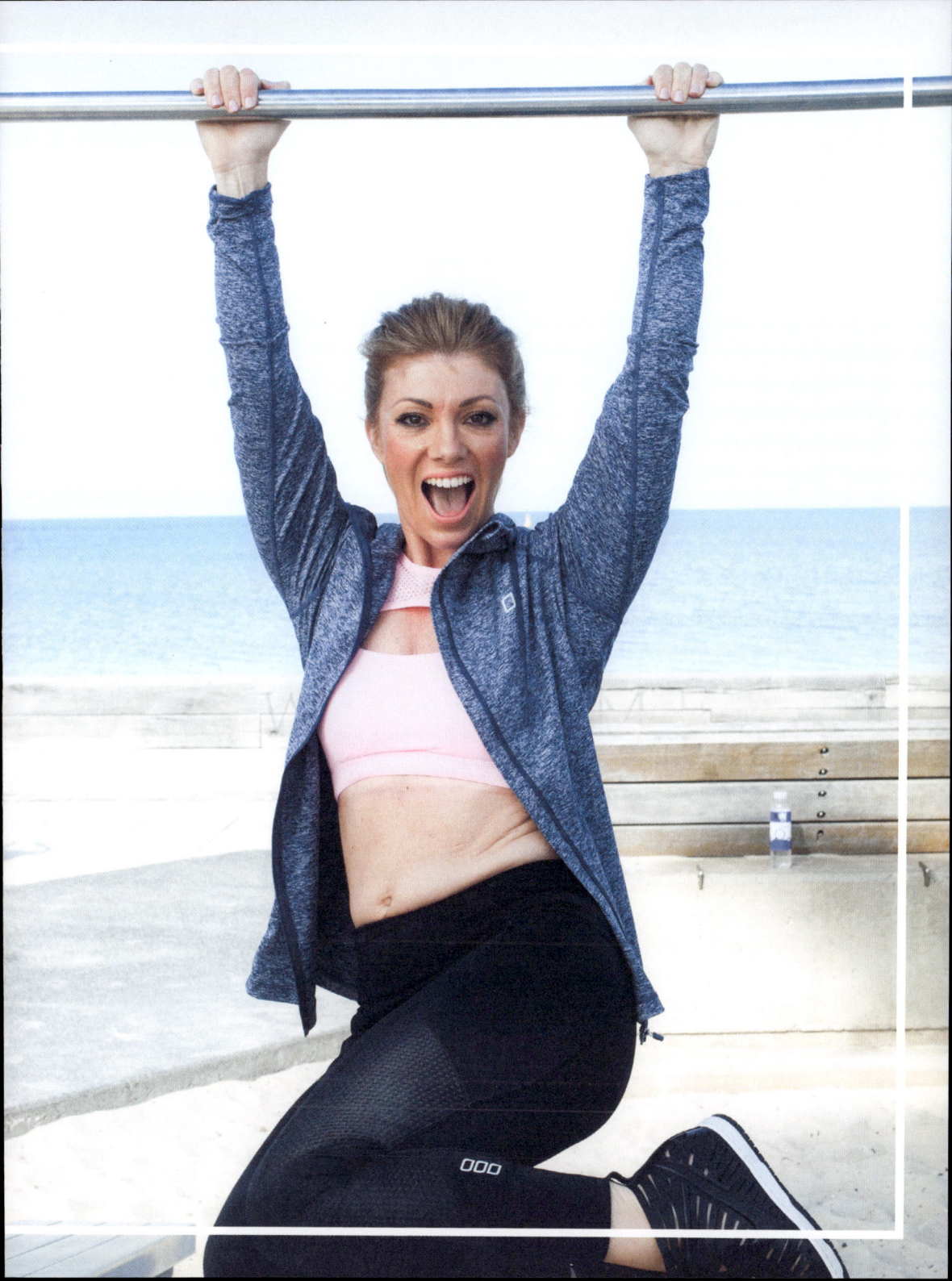

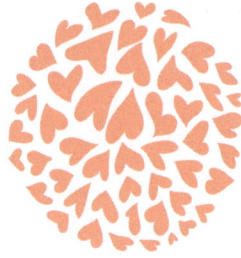

Using symptoms to empower you

YOU WILL LEARN ABOUT:

• inflammation • insulin resistance • gut health

We often loathe symptoms, probably because they are uncomfortable or, in more extreme cases, painful. I understand how frustrating that can be. But they are always a clue into the internal landscape of the body. Inflammation is a normal body response: it can show up as swelling after being wounded or when it gets a little out of control it can lead to issues like period pain or endometriosis and digestive issues, too. Inflammation isn't necessarily bad when it's under control. It's when it's combined with other factors that things can spiral.

In order to use symptoms to empower you, you must change your relationship with them.

Inflammation

We are all equipped to deal with inflammation in our body each and every day; however, some of us do a better job than others. First up, we need a body with a working inflammatory response. Inflammation serves a very important purpose – it is the release of special chemicals by the cells of our immune system that can trigger various types of healing as well as send out warning signs that things aren't ok. It also puts the body on alert by creating 'noise' to show other immune cells that help is needed, such as when we've been attacked by viruses, bugs or bacteria. It's your own defence system that is inbuilt; you don't need to do anything to trigger it, just like you don't need to do anything to blink – your body knows what to do automatically. The inflammatory response is important when we have an infection or have cut or hurt ourselves; however, what we don't want is the body to be in a constant state of alert, aka inflammation.

When inflammatory chemicals are out of control they can begin to cause damage to your cells and, over the long term, can be rather ruthless. It certainly isn't ideal to experience long-term inflammation in our body. This left untreated may damage our hormones. Since hormones are responsible for thousands of body processes (remember your hormones are your life hack) you may find symptoms to be wide and varied, ranging from issues with gut health right through to depression, painful periods or PCOS, to name a few of many. At the core of all hormone imbalance lies some kind of inflammation; the trick is pinpointing where it is stemming from.

CYTOKINES

Cytokines are the special chemical signals responsible for the entire inflammatory process released from your immune cells. Cytokines tell the rest of the body it's time to pull out the forces and fight like it's war and there's no tomorrow. For those with PCOS, you may find yourself with chronic low-grade inflammation since cytokines may be secreted constantly in low amounts, leading to a host of unwanted symptoms due to the ovaries being stimulated to create excess testosterone. What's more, this action also leads to insulin resistance as it goes to work on your fat cells.

KNOW THIS:

- Inflammation is often at the root of hormone imbalance. It may be the reason you experience period pain, acne or eczema. It's simply when the immune system is in overdrive.

- Inflammation can occur anywhere - your skin (acne or eczema), your uterus (i.e. endometriosis), your digestive system (bloating or pain).

- Inflammation can be a result of poor diet, lifestyle, environmental toxins, stress, your genetics and your emotions.

A WORD ON AUTOIMMUNITY

You may have heard of autoimmune illnesses where the immune system goes into overdrive and begins to produce antibodies against your body's own tissues (rather than against a virus or bacteria). This is a normal body function to fight infection (as we learnt when discussing UTIs) and our immune system should be able to respond correctly to what's being served up. It is, however, when this goes unchecked for a period of time and the immune system goes into overkill that there is even more inflammation. Many of the same chemicals that we see in inflammation are produced and potentially a few others thrown into the mix. It is these that can be harmful to the body. In many instances of hormone imbalance there are underlying autoimmune issues that need to be addressed and it can be useful to call upon your health professional to have you adequately tested for antibodies. This is something you may need to request as it isn't always procedure.

Tests

Tests you might like to request include Anti-TPO (Anti-Thyroid Peroxidase) and ANA (Anti-Nuclear Antibodies). Anti-TPO assesses the attack on the thyroid gland, which can be issues behind thyroid-related conditions (also associated with menstrual issues). ANA is a fundamental test for a variety of autoimmune conditions and celiac disease.

TREATING INFLAMMATION

A large portion of your inflammation stems from your digestive health – your gut, as mentioned, is the epicentre of your health and responsible for around 80% of your immune function. When the intestinal cells begin to lose strength, we can see leaky gut – when the intestinal barrier is no longer sealed and the contents of the intestine (including food, bacteria and chemicals) may essentially leak into the body. This isn't ideal and the body can certainly go into fight mode to do its job to rid itself of these things it sees as toxic. It can be this occurrence that triggers inflammation in your body and, depending on how your genes have blessed you, it can develop anywhere. Chances are, at the core of your health concerns is some inflammation.

Insulin resistance

Insulin resistance is often at the centre of your hormone issues. In your healthy body, insulin is secreted by the pancreas in response to blood sugar and is then sent to activate your cells for energy. When we are constantly at the pantry cupboard, eating our way through the day, our insulin levels may never drop and we can become desensitised to this normal body response. This means you may have extra blood sugar roaming in the blood that can cause damage, leading to type 2 diabetes, PCOS and more. Insulin loves to store fat as well, so even those of you who are trying to eat right might have problems losing weight and yes, you might even gain weight.

WHAT TO KNOW

- Pancreas releases insulin in response to blood sugar (after sweets and carbs). This is sent to activate cells to allow them to take glucose as fuel.
- Insulin encourages the body to store this energy as glycogen (it's one directional into the cells for immediate use or storage) for when energy is needed (mostly stored in the liver and muscles).
- High blood sugar is dangerous and can damage the liver, pancreas, brain, heart and eyes, and causes inflammation in the body.
- Once the liver is full and should blood sugar continue to be 'topped up', this excess energy needs a place to be stored.
- The liver takes the excess glucose and turns it into a special fat called triglycerides. Triglycerides are associated with weight gain due to fat storage.
- Women with PCOS often have high triglycerides, are insulin resistant and store excess fat.

In a healthy body insulin acts on the ovaries to produce testosterone, a precursor to other important hormones like oestrogen. But the rising testosterone (due to insulin) can totally affect your menstrual cycle and effectively pull the handbrake on your period and cycles. Over time, cells no longer respond to insulin, hence the name insulin resistance. It becomes a vicious cycle: the pancreas responds to rising sugar in the blood, producing more insulin, but the cells don't respond and so it roams the body like an underworld gang, causing havoc and affecting everything else around it.

A note about insulin and PCOS

Excess roaming insulin stimulates the ovaries to make more testosterone, which may be at the centre of your PCOS. We also now know that women with PCOS are much more prone to insulin resistance due to the genetic and inflammatory component of the condition. But it is not only women with PCOS who may have insulin resistance; it can be at the core, in some capacity, of most hormone imbalance.

MANAGING YOUR INSULIN

As a young woman it can be tricky to address insulin resistance but there is some great merit to diet and lifestyle in managing it. Here are my favourite suggestions:

Fasting

Just 12 hours of fasting can be enough to make your cells more sensitive to insulin. I suggest finishing up from food after dinner at night (making your last meal around 7 pm) and not eating again until 7 am. This will give you 12 hours overnight to allow your digestive system to do its job (your body likes to sleep, not digest, at 2 am) and help manage your blood sugar without upsetting your hormones. Do this for at least 3 days of the week – this is known as crescendo fasting. The way you approach 'fasting' overnight may change according to your condition but this is a safe way to approach it that won't impose on your hormones as they find their groove. **Instead of fasting all day, simply finish eating at 7 pm until 7 am on 2–3 non-consecutive nights per week.**

Supplements to consider

Vitamin D is crucial as it supports hormone balance and oestrogen regulation as well as healthy gut function. 1000 IU per day is my recommendation. If there is a family history of breast cancer, this is one supplement you are going to want to include no matter what. Research suggests that women who have adequate vitamin D are 80% less likely to develop breast cancer. **Inositol** is an extremely safe supplement that is insulin sensitising. **Berberine** is also an insulin sensitiser and supports healthy gastrointestinal function.

Diet

Diet plays a huge role. By the time you're finished with this book, you'll be a pro! Reducing dairy and sugar is a big factor in managing insulin resistance. **Check with your doctor before fasting, changing medications or taking supplements.**

Gut health

Your digestive system is the epicentre of your health as we've come to understand. Digestive health therefore counts most. Intestinal cells should provide a sealed barrier (the cells that make up the wall of your gut), protecting the bloodstream from contents of the intestine.

Food allergies and intolerances (for example, gluten) may provide particular insight into what is happening internally. Here's what may be playing out.

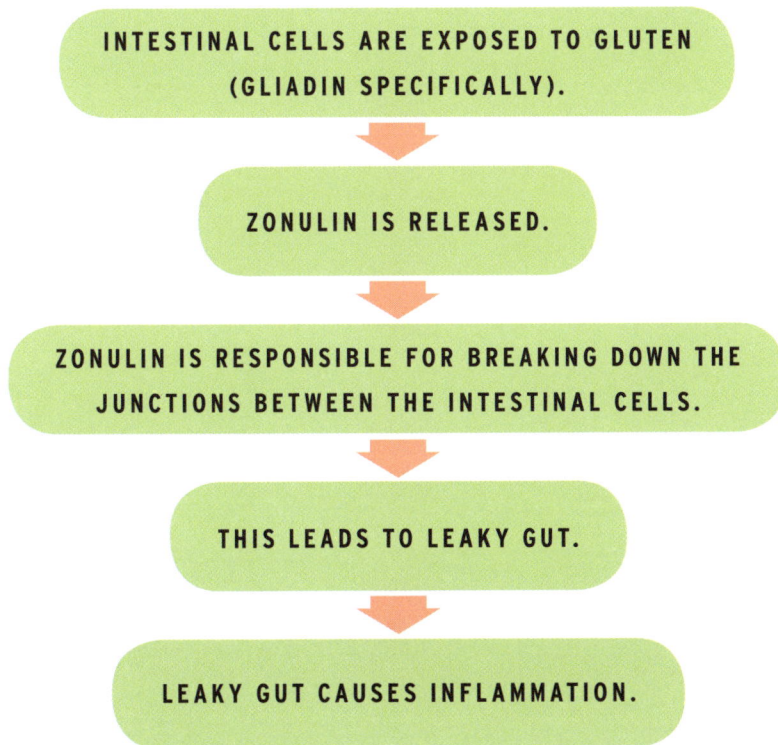

INTESTINAL CELLS ARE EXPOSED TO GLUTEN (GLIADIN SPECIFICALLY).

↓

ZONULIN IS RELEASED.

↓

ZONULIN IS RESPONSIBLE FOR BREAKING DOWN THE JUNCTIONS BETWEEN THE INTESTINAL CELLS.

↓

THIS LEADS TO LEAKY GUT.

↓

LEAKY GUT CAUSES INFLAMMATION.

LEAKY GUT SYNDROME:
HOW GLUTEN CAUSES GUT LEAKINESS

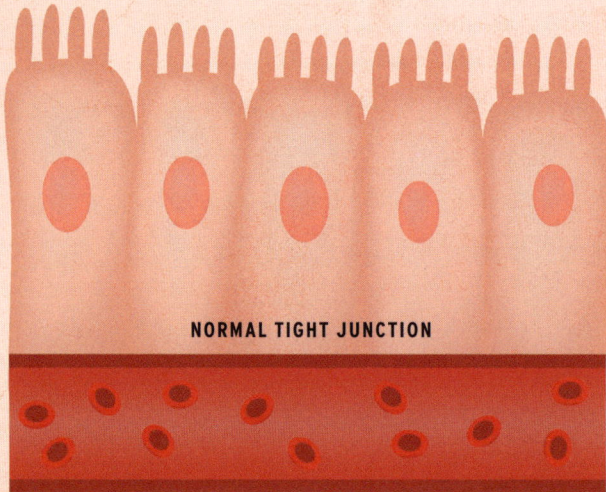

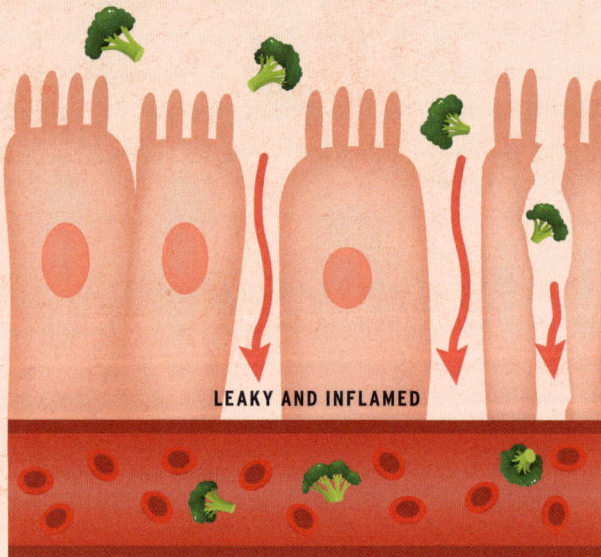

NORMAL TIGHT JUNCTION

LEAKY AND INFLAMED

As we've discussed, the microbiome and gut flora are equally important. Remember these are the essential life-giving bacteria that live in our digestive system and on us. We also know that these vital bacteria contain genes that make our own genes work. If there is overgrowth of unwanted or 'bad' bacteria, this function evidently is skewed and we may begin to experience a plethora of unwanted symptoms.

A WORD ON PREBIOTICS

As important as probiotics are prebiotics; they actually become more important in the role of constantly feeding good intestinal bacteria. If probiotics are the seeds to life, prebiotics are the fuel that allows the seeds to grow. Much like a seed needs sunlight, nutrient-rich soil, water and food, your gut bacteria needs to be fed the right things to continue to do its job. Prebiotics are simply foods we should have in our diet to achieve this. My favourite prebiotics and probiotics are:

Prebiotics

- Psyllium
- Slippery elm powder
- Asparagus
- Cooked onions (of any variety)
- Garlic
- Artichokes (all varieties)
- Bananas
- Barley
- Oats (Although they contain gluten, they can be good.)

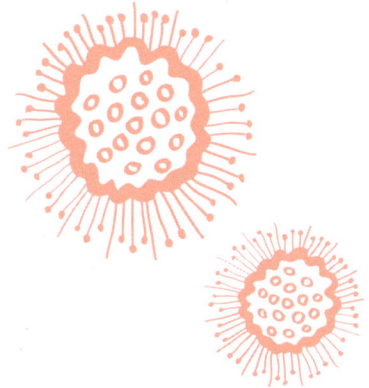

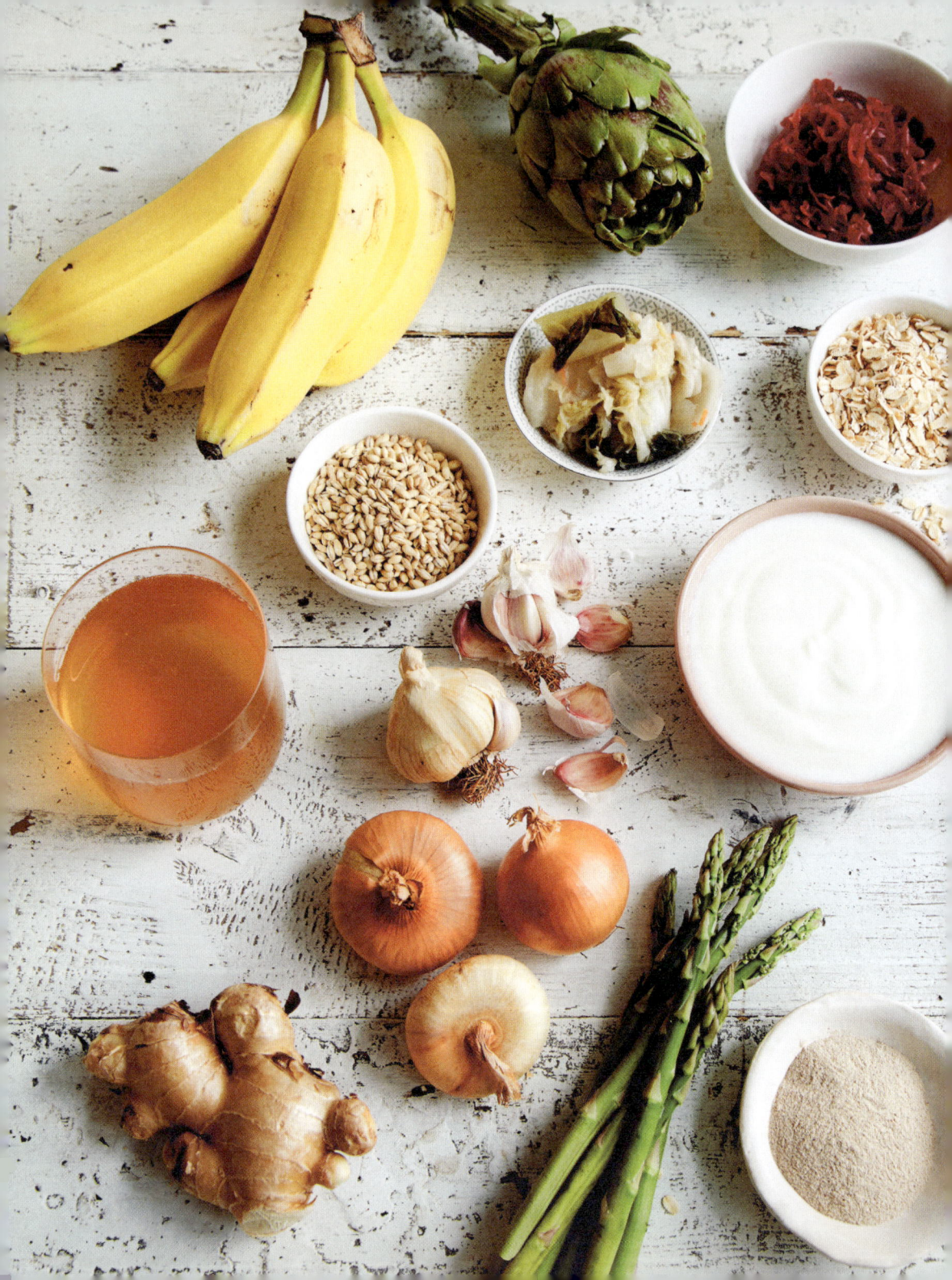

Probiotics

- Kombucha (fermented tea)
- Sauerkraut
- Fermented vegetables (sauerkraut/kimchi)
- Kefir yoghurt

A WORD ON PROBIOTICS

Probiotics are still essential and something I have my patients eat in small amounts, regularly. Less is definitely more when it comes to these foods. Too much and you may find yourself feeling out of sorts. For those who have never eaten such foods before, it's especially important to start slowly – $\frac{1}{2}$ teaspoon per day to start. There is a period of time when you begin taking probiotics when you can feel a little odd, sort of like you're getting a cold or flu. This is normal and temporary, and should never actually make flu status. It's known as 'die off' where the good bacteria are literally going to war with the not so good. Die off shouldn't last more than 2 weeks and for many, is very minimal. It's just good to be aware that if you do feel a bit odd, this is the reason.

Supplements

Supplements are available for prebiotics and probiotics as well as collagen or gelatin to address gut permeability. If supplements are your preference, that's totally fine; however, since looking after your gut health is a lifetime gig, I prefer to have patients incorporate these foods into their everyday regime. What's more, the wide variety of strains of bacteria we may get in a jar of sauerkraut outweighs what we would get in a supplement, just by the nature of the fermentation and how the process continues for as long as that jar of fermented vegetables sits in your fridge. It's a cheap and easy option; however, if that is a struggle, then of course supplements are the next best option. **The contents in supplements may vary between brands. Consult your healthcare practitioner for guidance and see your doctor if you experience side effects or discomfort.**

Sometimes supplements can be great for a more specific approach, such as if there is a particular diagnosed overgrowth or when something fast acting is required. Your healthcare practitioner is the best person to speak to about this in terms of the most appropriate approach. You can, however, safely invest in an over-the-counter probiotic to support your healthy gut best.

FOOD

To best treat gut permeability (to strengthen the junctions of the cells of the gut wall), we've seen that leaving out foods that lead to inflammation is the key. These typically are gluten, sugar and dairy (all the good stuff!). This will help you actually rebuild your gut without the distraction and chaos that these foods may cause. While these foods are on the 'out' list for a little while, it's during this time that we can best repair these cell junctions and gut integrity on the whole. This is done again via food and there are a few key players:

Collagen (found in gelatin) is key to assisting in this repair-and-rebuild phase and helps to strengthen the gut wall and address permeability. The best source is from slow-cooked meats, stews, broths, roasts and soups. Whenever meat is cooked over a period of time, the gelatin component found in the sinews and bones has an opportunity to make its way into the food and you reap the benefits.

Zinc is also excellent for supporting the cell junctions of the gut wall. For my vegetarian friends, you can consider using quercetin and glutamine 100 mg daily to assist in this process, too. This is particularly useful for those who don't eat meat, since the highest forms of collagen and gelatin are found in animals.

Treat the gut by avoiding certain foods for a while.

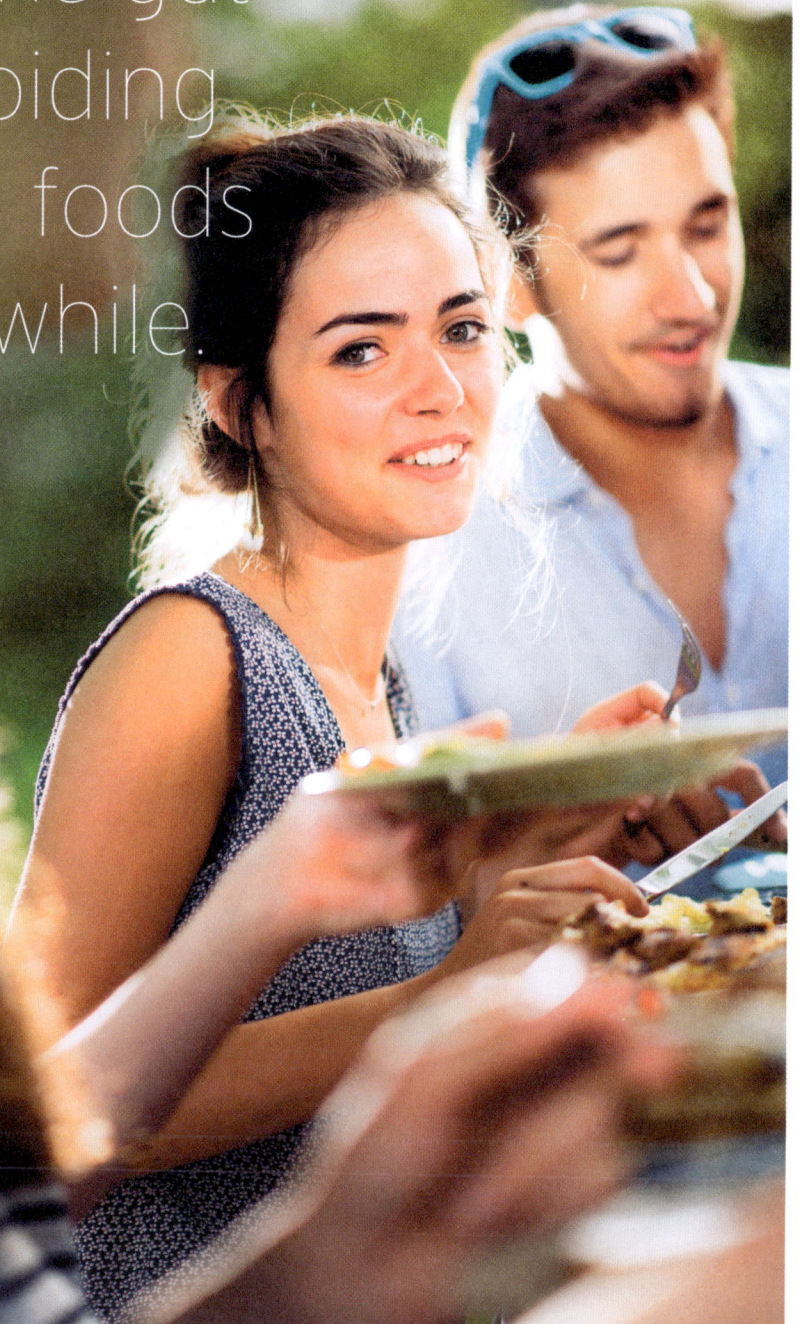

CHAPTER 6

Your options

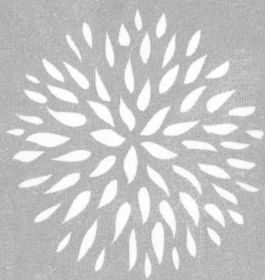

'There's always fear of the unknown where there's mystery.'

DAVID LYNCH

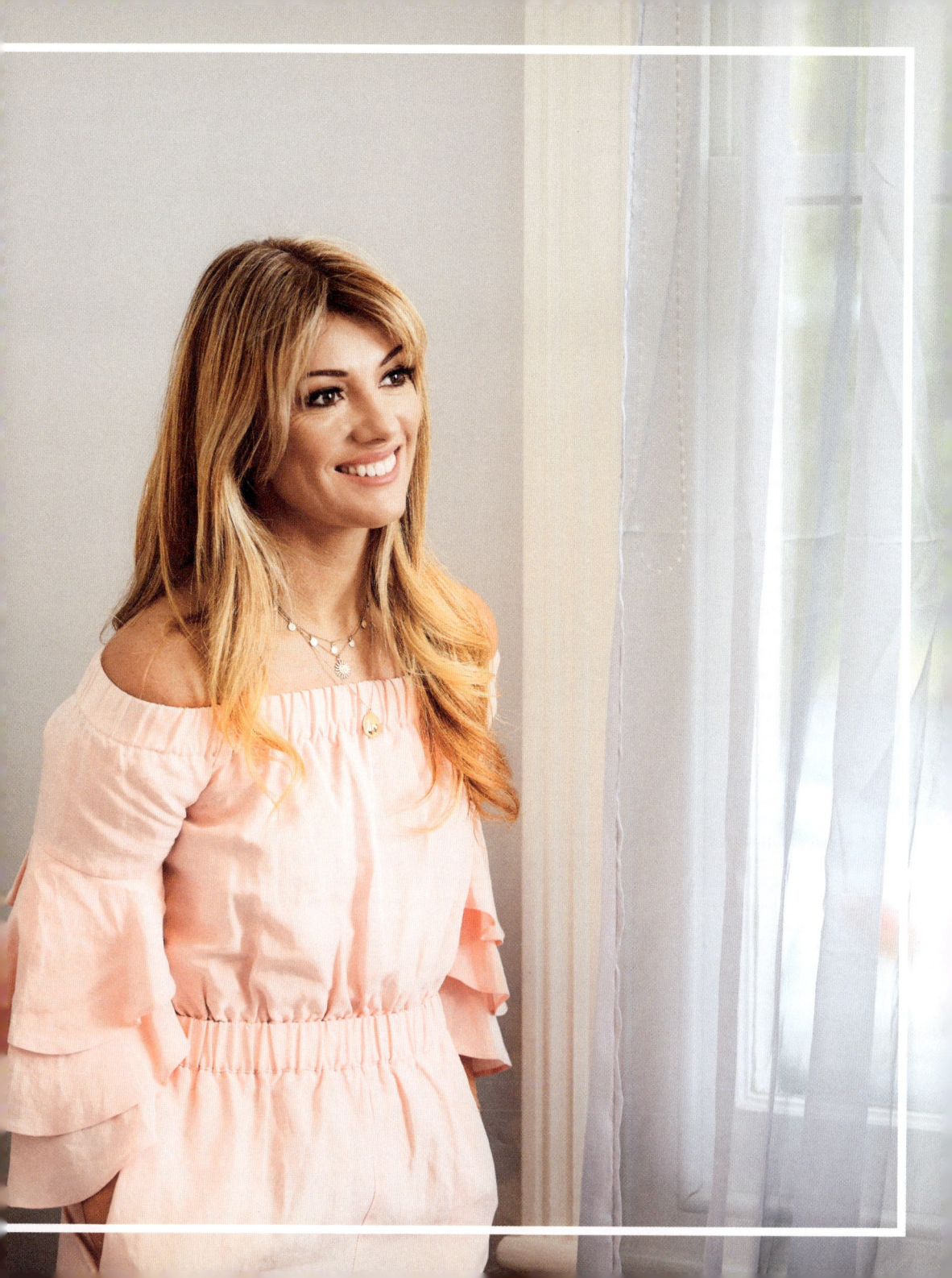

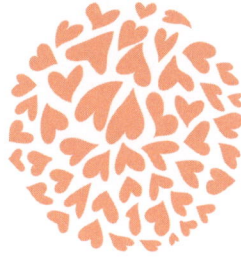

Finding the answers within us

YOU WILL LEARN ABOUT:

• diagnosis • testing • contraception

Once we understand a known 'problem' we can find a great solution. Knowledge frees us. Symptoms are clues into your internal world – what's important is that you use this as a guide. It's most important to remember, you do not need to suffer!

The mystery that comes with the unknown can be completely consuming.

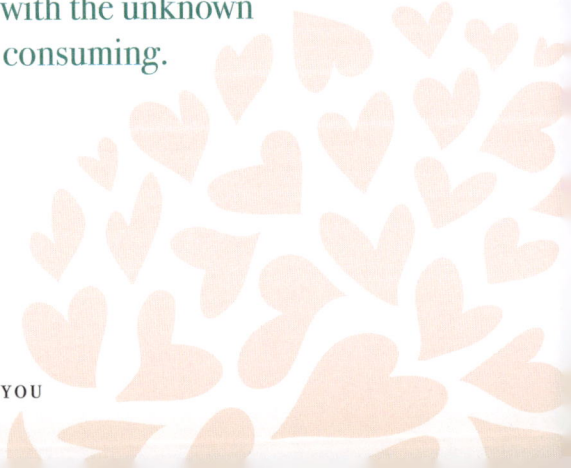

Diagnosis

Maybe you have a specific diagnosis of a particular condition or problem, prompted by symptoms. You started noticing some odd changes or that things weren't quite going to plan and you sought help from your doctor to get some answers. On the flip side, maybe you don't have any known issues. But at some point in your life, be it for yourself or for those around you that you love, you're going to be faced with not necessarily knowing what's actually going on internally and unless you are a doctor (and even then, we can't all know everything in any given moment), fear of the worst-case scenario kicks in.

Fear can take us one of two places. It can be your direct dial into action or it can be that you buy into the stress, which only creates more fear. But if your fear can be your strength, then it can be extremely useful. The trick is getting comfortable with facing fear front on and, once you've exercised this muscle a few times, you'll wonder why you never used its powerful energy before.

The mystery that comes with the unknown can be completely consuming. By nature, and I'd suggest also by conditioning of a world led by fear, most of us default to focusing on the worst-case scenario. It may be because of our love of drama or because we live in a constant state of stress. Whatever your innate (or learnt) response, we can generally do better.

As consumers, we love a diagnosis. We want to be able to label our problem. I once had a patient who had all the obvious signs of PCOS. She was slightly overweight, her periods were a mess on her calendar, she had acne and facial hair, and her emotions were all over the place. She came to me and I began to treat what I saw, not through testing (yet) but via her very clear signs and symptoms. Two weeks later she busted into my clinic completely devastated by her recent PCOS diagnosis. I sat her down and asked her why this made her so upset and her conclusion was that she now had PCOS and everything she had heard about the condition was trouble. She feared the worst. I explained to her that the 'label' she now had didn't really change much, it was just a name for a bunch of symptoms we were already treating. Through her tears she looked at me and I could see her relief. I could show her she was buying into the 'label' and that she wasn't PCOS at all, she was somebody who *had* PCOS.

We can very rapidly become, or step into being, our problem. That is, when we are given our diagnosis we buy in. The truth is, more than likely nothing has changed, yet we all of a sudden attach and cling to the problem as if it is a liferaft.

You are not your problem. Just like you are not a fingernail. You, of course, have fingernails but you are not a walking fingernail.

Perhaps we love to cling to the label because it justifies our problems or symptoms. When we can blame it on hormones or genetics, we may feel a sense of relief that it isn't our fault and I'm here to say that, knowingly of course, it isn't your fault at all.

But getting comfortable with accepting that the label is our destiny is where things need to change. Generally our genetics, as we've learnt, dictate what could possibly show up but equally it can be all the other things going on in our lives that contribute to turning on or off the reactions that play out inside of us. So for example, you may be predisposed to PCOS; however, you don't have symptoms of PCOS because nothing in your life to date has pushed your body far enough out of its natural state of homeostasis (your body's own equilibrium switch that likes to keep things in balance) to flick on those symptoms. What this means is we can't use our genetics as an excuse for our issues because we can lead our body back to a better state of balance and with this comes fewer symptoms. In fact, when you can identify the stressor or driver of the problem, you can generally treat it with great success. The trick is being able to work out what this is and begin to act accordingly.

So you see, getting your diagnosis isn't the be all and end all. Of course, I'm not encouraging you to ignore your symptoms, they should always be explored, but should your doctor find something is up, most often than not it is a treatable condition and leading your body back to a state of wellness isn't always as hard as we've been led to believe.

Getting back to the fear again. When we make decisions based on fear we can wind up on the back of a buggy being dragged about the place. To me, education is the greatest gift. When you can understand your health and get a grasp of what might not be working properly and why, the game changes. Making educated decisions that are driven by being informed is without doubt the most empowering experience. Having the right questions to ask your doctor and feeling like you have all the facts and information can remove the fear instantly. Couple this with being able to tap into what intuitively feels good is the trifecta. Because nobody can actually know your body better than you.

<blockquote>
Nobody can know your body better than you.
You are the only person who can know how
you feel in the skin you're in.
</blockquote>

We often hope that our healthcare professional will give us the magic pill to fix the problem, yet sadly no such thing exists. There is, however, one sure thing you can do to take your health where you want it to go and that is to understand why it's misbehaving. It isn't just doing it to punish you; there is always a good reason.

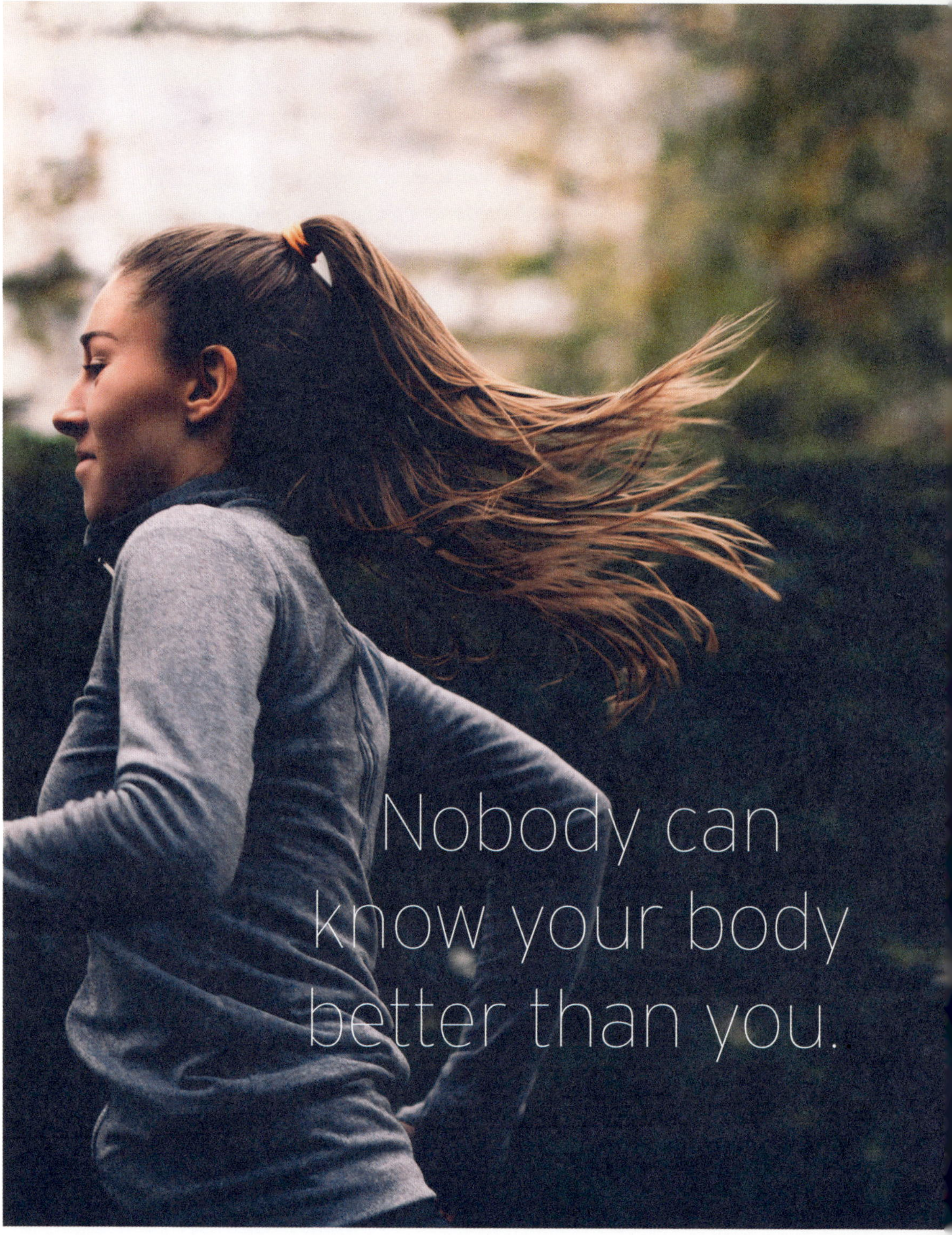

Nobody can
know your body
better than you.

Testing

Testing can be a great start to understand your body a bit better. It creates an excellent benchmark to also be able to compare progress (or lack of, too). However, over my time as a practitioner I've come to learn that putting all of your eggs into that basket can be a disaster.

I once had a patient who came to me after being diagnosed by her doctor with adrenal fatigue, which is an issue that can arise after extreme stress, where the adrenals are so overworked they begin to burn out. This diagnosis was based only on her most recent blood test conducted by her doctor. He made the call, she was devastated, and came to me for some help since Western medicine doesn't offer any real solutions as it stands for adrenal fatigue. When I consulted with her, I couldn't see any stand-out symptoms to support this diagnosis. Her sleep was good, her appetite was fine and her periods were regular. Her skin looked bright and she was generally happy.

It was apparent to me that the blood test was telling us something that wasn't confirmed by her signs. So I asked her what happened before the blood test that may have affected the results. She went on to tell me how much she feared blood tests and how they made her worried, nervous and stressed. I concluded that based on this, her cortisol potentially wasn't an ongoing issue but had responded to her stress in the lead up to the blood test. Nothing more. I never needed to treat her, she was generally happy and healthy, but it shows that sometimes our test results aren't always reflective of what's truly going on. This is especially true for blood tests, which aren't often a good indicator.

Blood tests generally reflect levels of various existing factors or markers within the body. They don't tell us how your body is using such things. So for example, your progesterone levels according to your blood tests suggest that everything is well within range. However, if for some reason your cells aren't taking or using progesterone properly, this may explain why your results look ok but your cycles are a disaster. This is the downside of blood testing.

In clinic, I prefer to use systems that test for how your hormones are being used in your body. These tests are relatively new but tell us a lot about the internal landscape. One example is the DUTCH test (Dried Urine Test for Comprehensive Hormones). Saliva testing is also great. The difference here is that these tests aren't generally covered by health insurance and you'll be out of pocket to have them done.

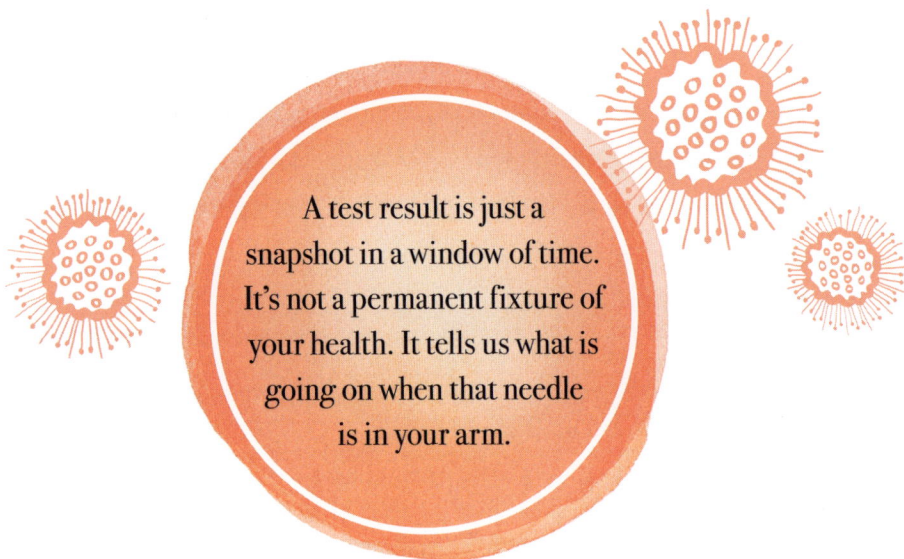

> A test result is just a snapshot in a window of time. It's not a permanent fixture of your health. It tells us what is going on when that needle is in your arm.

In any case, use your test results as a guide, not an end point. There are always improvements and changes to be made. Allow your test to motivate you towards better health and know that nothing is permanent.

Contraception

Contraception, or birth control, comes in a number of forms: pills, devices, procedures. Some contain hormones, some don't. All have advantages and disadvantages.

SYNTHETIC HORMONE CONTRACEPTION

The pill

If I had a tally for the number of women I see post pill that say to me 'if I had known it was going to mess with my body this much, I never would have taken it in the first place', I'd need shares in a paper mill to record them all. It's only now, some 50 odd years on since the pill was first released, that we are realising it may actually cause a few problems with our hormones. In fact, all synthetic hormone contraceptives do at some level, and if you're having problems, a different brand with different levels of hormones may work better for you, although I'd still advocate for you to get to the root cause of your hormone imbalance. Let's give them a quick rundown.

The pill also severely disrupts healthy gut function, which affects the body's ability to absorb vitamins and minerals. Because of this reason alone, many women find themselves totally affected by the pill. In my experience, even if you aren't seeing effects, they tend to catch up with you purely because your body doesn't like running on empty.

As a practitioner I certainly don't judge women who decide to take synthetic hormone contraceptives; however, I do like to make them aware just how many of their complaints may be easily alleviated without synthetic hormones. The number one problem with this synthetic contraception is that when it is prescribed, very little information about what the pill does is ever given to a patient.

FACTS ON THE 'PILL'

- The pill makes us temporarily infertile because it is designed to do so. It stops our hormones from cycling, stopping ovulation and therefore the period.

- It may upset our hormone balance and in many instances, our bodies may have trouble getting back on track. It all depends on the individual.

- We do not have a period on the pill – we experience a withdrawal bleed.

- The pill is the most commonly prescribed drug worldwide for birth control and is used to treat a host of conditions from premenstrual tension, ovulation pain right through to conditions like endometriosis.

- Unfortunately, it isn't a solution to PCOS or endometriosis since solutions fix problems. The pill is a temporary 'fix' that may provide you with some relief and a chance to take a breath but it isn't a long-term fix. If only.

- According to Professor Erik Odeblad, who has studied the cervix for 40 years, the pill degenerates the crypts (the small areas in the cervix that secrete discharge and mucus) essential for conception. Without fertile mucus, the sperm can't reach the egg.

- Side effects include nausea, depression, breast pain, migraines and low libido (the latter I find ironic ... if you are on the pill for contraceptive reasons, but you can't entertain the thought of jumping your partner and getting between the sheets, it's kinda defeating the purpose IMO).

- Research conducted by Marie Stopes on women, contraception and unplanned pregnancy in 2008 suggested the pill can make for a very unsettled baby and mother, should a woman fall pregnant shortly after coming off the pill.

- According to the book, *The Pill* by Jane Bennett and Alexandra Pope, the pill alters our senses and skews our radar when it comes to attracting a suitable (compatible – when it comes to baby making) partner as it alters our pheromones (the chemicals we release into the environment that others sense, which attracts us to people).

- It doesn't protect against STIs.

Implanon (birth control implant)

The implanon is a plastic rod which contains progesterone and it is inserted just under the skin of the upper arm by your doctor. It's said to be more than 99% effective and, like the mirena or the copper IUD, it needs to be removed by your doctor.

FACTS ABOUT THE IMPLANON

- It works by stopping ovulation like the pill (OCP), thickening the cervical mucus and thinning the uterine lining.
- Many women experience amenorrhea while the implanon is in place (no periods).
- Spotting and bleeding is considered a common side effect.
- There can be complications with insertion and, while it's not common, the rod can migrate and move from the arm.
- Weight gain and acne are also commonly reported side effects.
- There is no protection against STIs.

Depo Provera (injection)

Depo Provera is a brand name for a slow-release hormone like progesterone that is injected into the buttocks or upper arm by a doctor. It is about 99.8% effective as a contraceptive.

FACTS ABOUT DEPO PROVERA

- It lasts about 3 months before the next injection is due.
- It can stop periods after 2-3 injections and ovulation ceases (the ovaries don't release eggs).
- It can take a long time to restart ovulation and periods normally once the injections cease. It is not suitable for women who want to become pregnant within 12 months.
- It may cause side effects such as fluid retention, spotting and weight gain. Once the injection has been given, the hormone cannot be removed.
- There is no protection against STIs.

The mirena

The mirena subscribes to the same concept as the copper IUD – in fact they are both IUDs with one difference. The mirena also contains hormones.

FACTS ON THE MIRENA

- It's a plastic T-shaped device. In the stem is a storage compartment containing hormones which are slowly released – the same that you will find in the OCP.
- The mirena may be suggested as being better than the pill because it is a lower dose compared to the OCP.
- The direct release of hormones into the womb acts in several ways. It increases the thickness of the cervical mucus, making implantation much more difficult. The IUD also thins the uterine lining, making implantation very difficult and for some women the mirena stops ovulation altogether.
- There is no protection against STIs.

Is the mirena better than the pill?

Many doctors will advocate for the mirena over the pill because it doesn't rely on you needing to take it every day, but unlike the pill, you need to have it removed if you want out. To me, both come with pros and cons.

Hormone contraceptives from the perspective of your gut health all come with similar effects. Many women report to me they bleed the entire month round with the mirena. It does leave me scratching my head – if you're using it for contraceptive purposes but you can never have sex because you're always bleeding ... what's the point? The mirena is commonly used to help manage conditions like PCOS and endometriosis. There is also the very real chance that the mirena is too big for a uterus that has never been pregnant.

NON-HORMONAL CONTRACEPTION

The copper IUD

This is an IUD like the mirena, with one main difference. The copper IUD doesn't contain hormones.

I don't have a favourite form of contraception mostly because they can come with a monster list of side effects, complications and troubles. But granted, I do only see women who have found themselves in trouble after using them and I'm assured there are millions of women reaping the benefits without too many issues that they are aware of or have not yet associated with synthetic hormones. The copper IUD (Intrauterine Device) is one many women turn to because it doesn't contain 'synthetic' hormones and I guess if you had to twist my arm, it would be for this reason the only one I'd advocate for – that doesn't mean it comes without complications.

FACTS ON THE COPPER IUD

- The copper IUD is a small intrauterine device that is placed inside the uterus to prevent pregnancy. The copper coil, which is wrapped around the IUD itself, releases ions into the surrounding fluids. This impairs the mobility of sperm like some kind of superhero magnetic force. The copper IUD is said to be around 99% effective and can keep working for up to 10 years (some suggest up to 20 years).

- The IUD also works as it changes the thickness of the uterine lining, affecting implantation. There are several theories around this – none of which have been 100% proven.

- Heavier and more painful periods are very common with a copper IUD.

- Infections are more common for women who have an IUD. There is a really high chance of infection developing in the first 20 or so days after insertion. Infection can lead to issues, such as infertility, Pelvic Inflammatory Disease (PID), scarring or damage, be it from the IUD itself or from a sexually transmitted illness.

- Women who have IUDs are also said to have an increased risk of ectopic pregnancies and miscarriage.

- IUDs do not offer protection from STIs, which can have the same ramifications as those I've mentioned for Pelvic Inflammatory Disease (PID).

Cervical cap and diaphragm

Fitted inside the woman by the woman, cervical caps and diaphragms prevent the sperm from reaching the egg. The cervical cap is the more modern version of the diaphragm. Both the cervical cap and the diaphragm sit over the cervix. The benefit of the cervical cap is that it can be fitted up to 6 hours prior to intercourse. There's no protection against STIs.

Condoms

Condoms provide an extremely effective barrier to prevent sperm making its way to the possible released egg to prevent pregnancy.

While condoms are used to prevent pregnancy, they are also effective in protecting against STIs – something that none of the other contraceptives do. This is extremely important for long-term health and wellbeing.

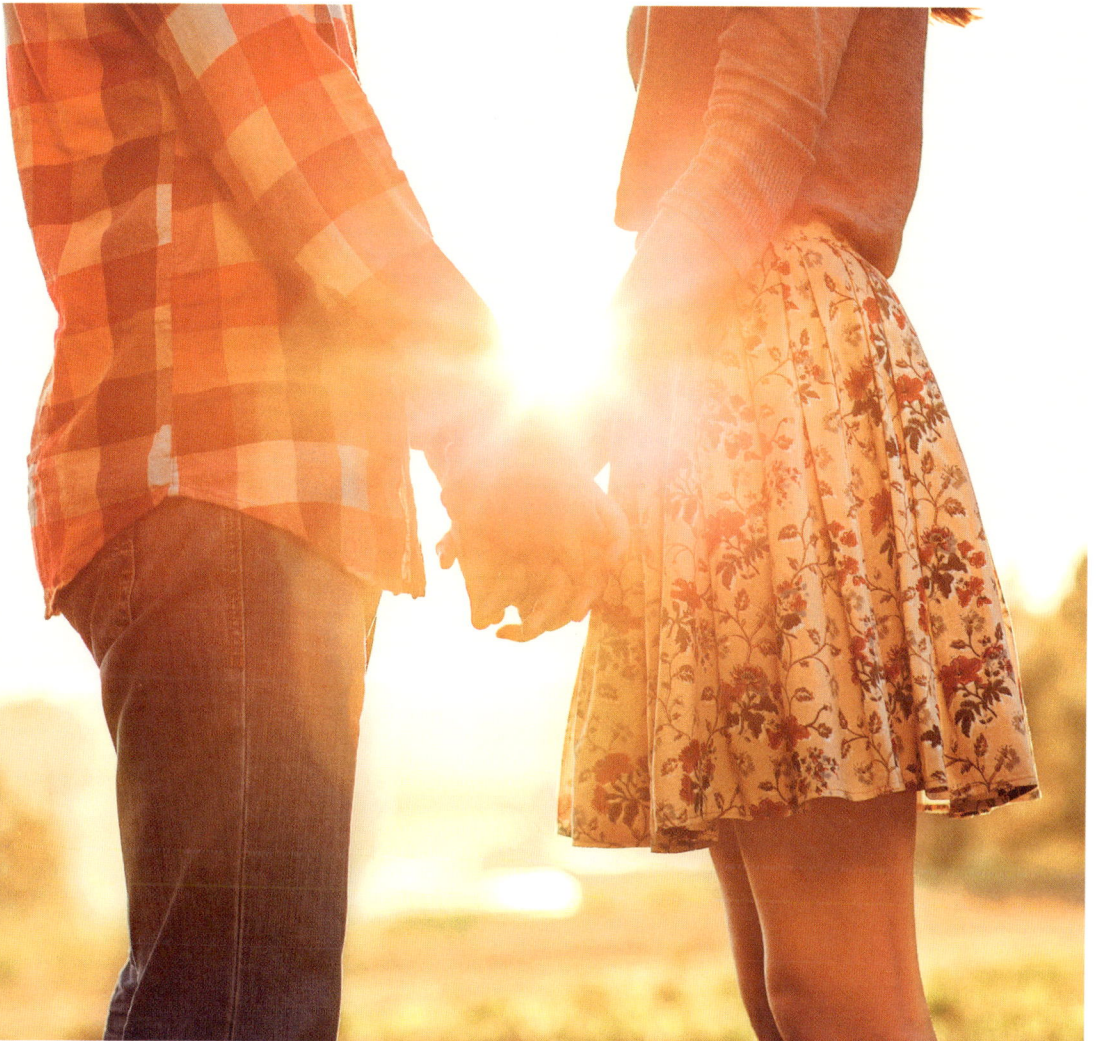

CHAPTER 7

Your wellbeing

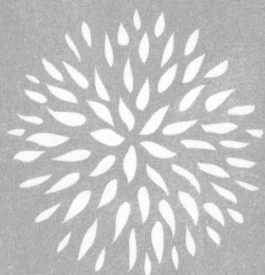

Beauty begins the moment
you decide to be yourself.

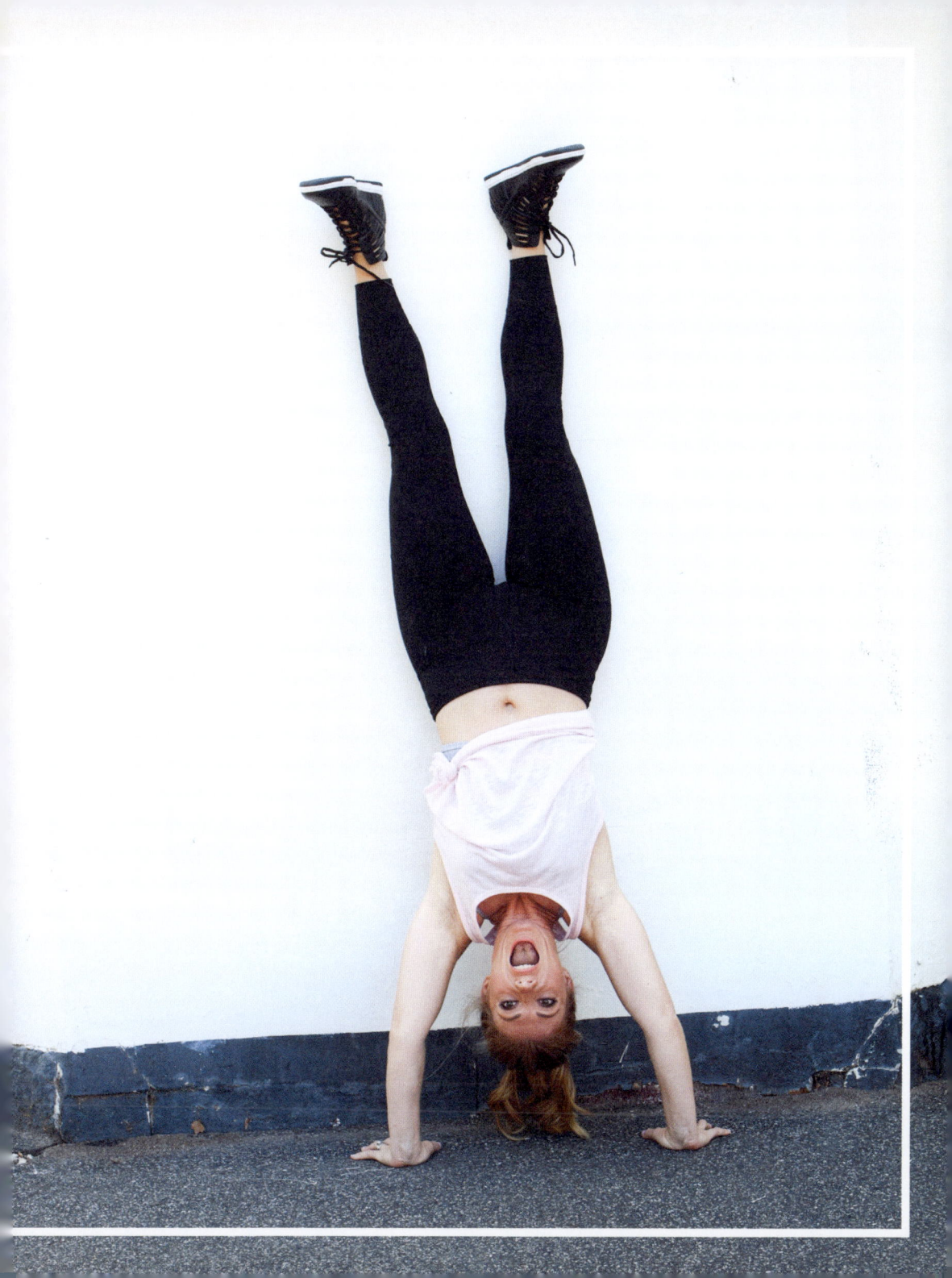

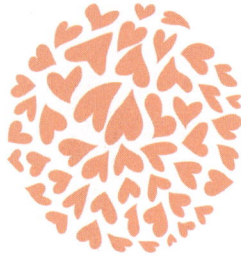

Feeling good more often

The four pillars of wellbeing are sleep, managing stress, moving your body well and being social. Tapping into this can really help you to be productive and feel healthy, too. Sleep is the elixir of health and should be an absolute priority.

Sleep

When researching this book I was totally floored to learn that an estimated 50% of the population are sleep deprived, or at best have circadian rhythms that are out of sync with their natural environment. I'm fairly sure all of you can relate to being tired or sleep deprived, possibly as recently as yesterday. Our circadian rhythm is what is said to make us want to sleep when it gets dark and leads us to wake when it gets light. This is a beautiful example of how our environment has a huge influence on our day-to-day life and health.

Within the circadian rhythm there are two factors to consider: the circadian clock and our sleep-wake homeostatic process. The circadian clock is what is cued from daylight or activities that may keep us awake and the sleep-wake homeostatic process is the accounting of the amount of sleep experienced in recent days, kind of like your sleep bank and much like your savings account.

> Your body knows when to rest and sleep.
> It's our ability to fight against it that
> can land us in a world of trouble.

Your body is always on a constant highway towards balance, which is a knee-jerk reaction to deficiency or debt. It is said that people with disturbed circadian cycles are more likely to develop mental and physical disorders, as well as sleep disorders as a direct hit from lack of sleep. These same people are more likely to also experience metabolic syndrome (the name given to a group of symptoms that increase the risk of heart disease, stroke and diabetes) and gastrointestinal or Glycemic Index (GI) issues, all because lack of sleep is stressful. When you can't sleep or don't sleep well, be it by choice or environment, every single cell in your body reacts.

SLEEP DEPRIVATION

Sleep deprivation, including insomnia, increases the risk of emotional disorders, cancer, brain problems, heart attack and heart disease, and even death. Obesity and diabetes are also more likely. **When we are sleep deprived we may be in a pre-diabetic state, making us feel hungry even though we've already eaten.**

Sleep deprivation also increases the risk of injury and poor decision-making; it sees us put ourselves in positions that we wouldn't entertain in our more 'sane' and nourished mind. Sleep deprivation, I say, is therefore quite possibly making us crazy!

When I dug further into research on sleep deprivation, I found the most recent findings pointed towards brain detoxification and how lack of sleep is upsetting our hormones – a game changer!

The solution is pretty simple – we need more sleep. We can create better sleeping habits (because apparently, it's about consistency when it comes to sleep) or at least look into why we aren't sleeping to get answers about our overall health. Sleep hygiene is just as important as food and if you think you can get away with less, think again.

Truthfully, you can never get back sleep that you lose.

If sleep is an issue, it's important to look at why: what is affecting sleep. Usually it is stress of some kind.

Sleep hygiene – habits to help you sleep better

- Sleep hygiene refers to a 'clean' sleeping environment and your bedtime routine.
- Make sure everything around you is in check – including the air you breathe and clean bedding.
- Rid your sleeping environment of Electromagnetic Fields (EMFs) and bright lights to help create a space that your body is ready to rest in.
- Introduce your favourite relaxing essential oils to help you sleep better.
- Use the moments before your sleep to check in and find three things you are grateful for from the day. This practice is said to have a profound impact on our emotional wellbeing and helps create a more positive start to the next day ahead.

A good sleeping environment has an enormous impact on the quality of our sleep.

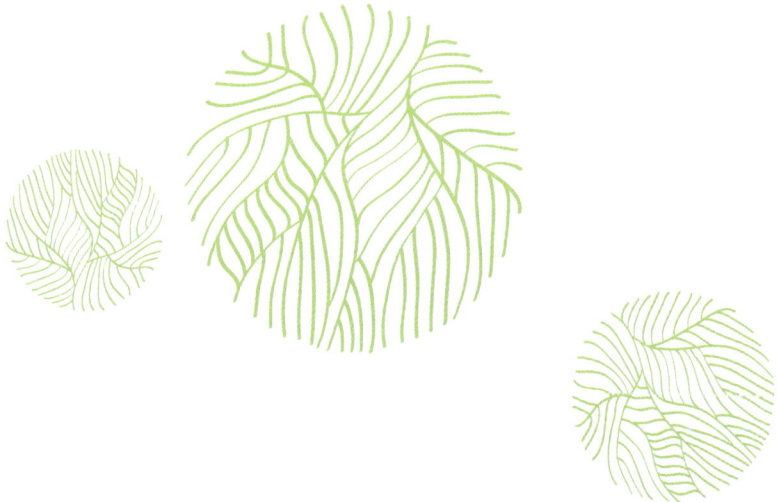

Stress

Stress sets off a chain of events in the body, decreases gut function, increases inflammation, interrupts sleep and upsets our hormones terribly. In fact, most modern illnesses can be linked back to stress of some kind. But stress can be many things; it's not just about being busy or having to meet a due date under pressure. Stress can be eating subaverage food, thinking unkind thoughts or not dealing with emotions when they arrive. Stress may also be your liver not working properly or your bowels being backed up. It can be stressful to look in the mirror every morning and say unkind things to yourself or hold a grudge against a loved one. Stress can be so many varied factors. Stress triggers the production of cortisol and adrenaline (your stress hormones), which severely disrupt the production of other hormones, especially progesterone and serotonin. Lack of serotonin can be an issue as it leads to food cravings and causes you to churn through magnesium faster than you can keep up. Magnesium is one of the key players in balanced hormones, too. But what's more, magnesium is necessary to produce serotonin and the vicious cycle continues. This is just one example of what stress can do.

Everything you've been learning in this book is ticking boxes in moving towards your 'less stressed self', but there are a few really simple additions you can add to your regimen that can be instant stress relievers.

- Read. It immediately relieves stress by up to 86%, according to a study by psychologist Dr David Lewis.
- Tea (here it is again). It lowers stress by up to 54% (concluded in the same study).

- Pump up the tunes. Listening to music lowers stress by up to 61%.
- Affirm. Use your affirmations to remind yourself that you choose ease today.

These are all wonderful short-term stress 'fixers'. Evidently, more long-term stress may involve a change of situation, removing yourself from stressful situations, friendships or workplaces. But ultimately recognising where your stress is coming from is the key to better managing it.

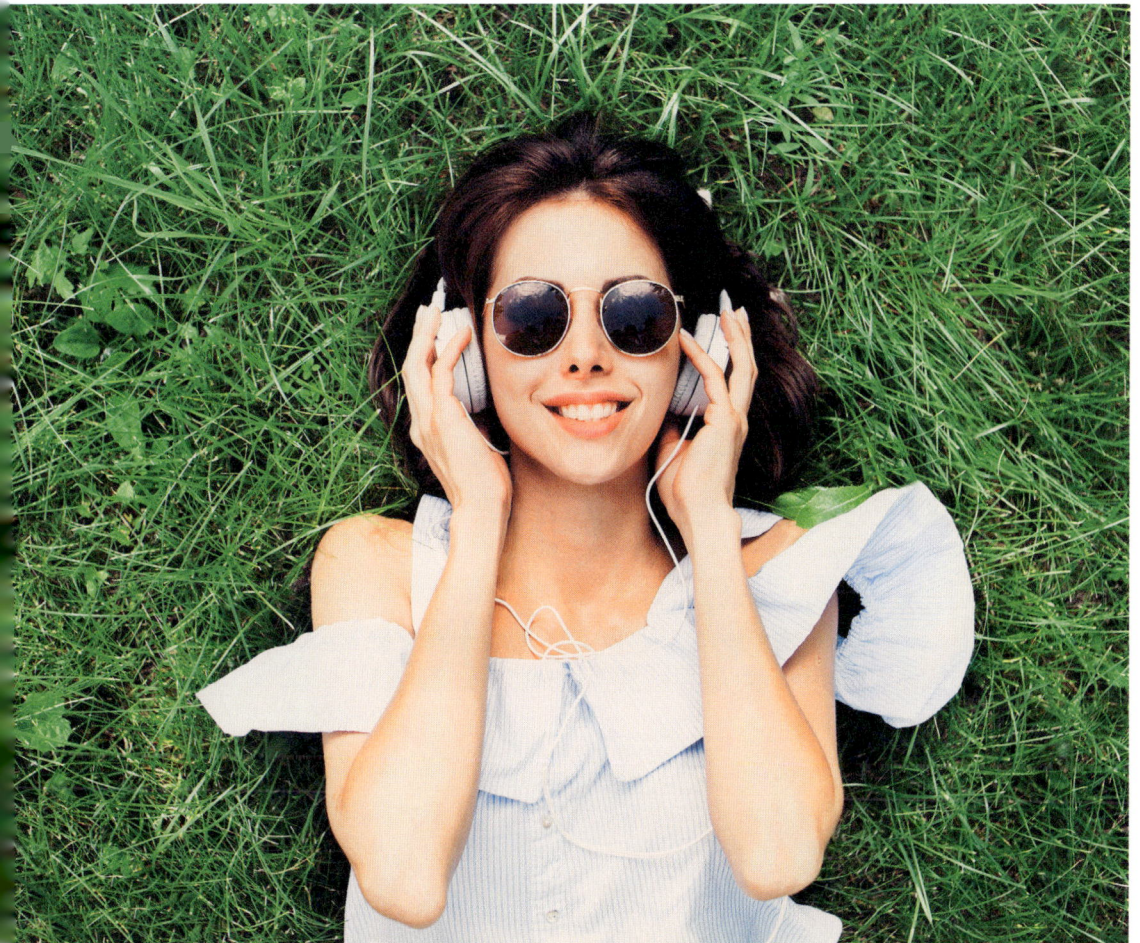

Exercise

Movement is extremely important as part of a healthy body. When we move, we naturally massage our lymph (our toxin removal system) so it can do its job; exercise helps us move excess stress hormones through the body and keeps our muscles and tendons conditioned. But the benefits of exercise in terms of our feel-good hormones are equally important. We once thought exercise was the key to healthy weight and, while movement is indeed important, weight management is far less about exercise and more about balancing the whole package.

It's important to move your body in such a way that it not only fits in with your cycle, but fits in with how you are feeling on any given day. Varied exercise is best and moving in a way that our body is designed to mechanically move is important – all muscle groups should be moved consistently. Gymnastics is a good example of a sport or exercise regimen where all muscle groups are exercised, whereas some weight-lifting routines isolate muscle groups.

When you activate your core and engage all muscle groups, you support healthy metabolism too.

Acts like pulling and pushing help to activate all of the muscle groups at the one time. You might consider sports that take this into consideration or that use your whole body, like swimming, hiking, surfing or rock climbing.

Weight training and low body weight can place huge stress on the body, which may contribute to stress and hormone imbalance. I always recommend short, sharp bursts of exercise rather than gruelling and lengthy workouts. I love incidental exercise and activities that are more about enjoying life but the trick is to find what works for you and movement that you love (not what you loathe).

Over-exercising, especially when our hormones are still finding their groove, is being researched more than ever and we now see a link between hormone imbalance and young athletes. Very often the menstrual cycle can be affected by high-intensity exercise or weight loss and it is important to explore this as soon as you see any changes. If you skip more than three menstrual cycles (and your cycles have previously been regular), it's much easier to fix early on than later in life.

REMEMBER

- Aim to move your body at least 20 minutes three times per week.

- Choose movement that you like – you're more likely to do it!

- Use movement as a time to get what you need. Want to be more social, walk with a friend or join a team. Need a little more downtime, pop in the earphones and enjoy the peace!

- Remember to take it easy around menstruation – listen to what your body is asking for and adjust where appropriate.

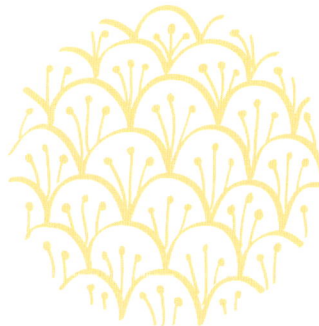

Socialising

Believe it or not, being social is a huge part of creating happy hormones. Spending time with the people you love boosts oxytocin (the feel-good hormone). The tricky part is, when we are feeling low, the last thing we might feel like doing is spending time with our favourite people; our innate reaction is to retract and retreat. This can become rather a trap because if we're feeling low and we continue to avoid family and friends, the cycle continues.

As humans, we are innately social beings and we perform at our best when we are interacting and connecting with others. It has been proven that spending time with the people you love most changes the neurotransmitter and circuit activity in the brain, which may assist in decreasing stress, depression and anxiety, and help increase the good 'feels'.

The release of oxytocin also supports the release of serotonin (your feel-good neurochemical) and interestingly helps you control your emotions since it calms the fear centre of your brain (the amygdala). Being social doesn't just have to be heading out with your bestie; you may choose to pick up the phone, chat on social media or email and text your favourite people – those people who help you be a better person. Anything less won't do and releasing toxic relationships is part of being happy and healthy, although it is easier said than done. Here are a few ways to boost your feel-good hormones:

• Participate in a regular activity with a friend. Play a team sport or meet up to walk around the block a few times a week. It doesn't have to be fancy, just regular.

- Get a massage. Massaging and touching helps release endorphins such as serotonin and dopamine, which helps keep a handle on cortisol, too. It also helps you sleep better!
- Spend time in nature. Get out in the sunshine, walk through the trees, take your shoes off and let your soles touch the earth. It can be very grounding and it helps you relax and reconnect with yourself, too.
- Grab a hug. A gentle, warm long hug helps release oxytocin. Steal a hug off friends, family or anybody who might be willing! Plus it makes you feel wonderful.

You can only change your own life by choosing to be part of it.

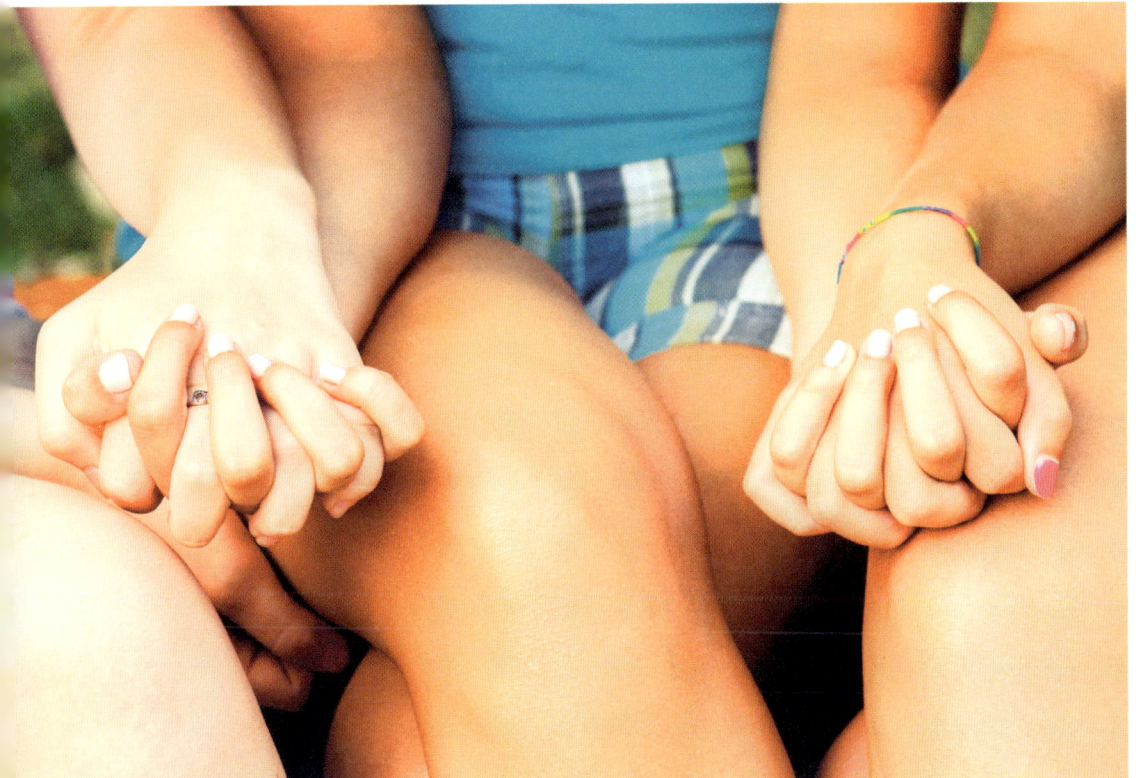

WORKSHEET: **FRIENDSHIPS**

Maybe you have toxic friendships that are constantly draining your oxytocin. It might be time to assess just how much of an influence negative people might be having on your life. If you feel down and out by being around certain people, maybe they aren't actually your people. All of us go through ups and downs, but if your friends are literally draining your spirit, it might be time to work out how to manage the situation better. After all, it's up to you to create the life that you deserve.

These people tend to be a little crafty, maybe talk about themselves a lot (and never about you) or possibly they are always having a crisis or gossiping about others (a key trait). I'm not here to say you need to leave them upstream without a paddle, that wouldn't make you feel great, but stepping back may be the difference between keeping you in a perpetual state of stress or stepping into your greatness.

To really assess this, ask yourself a few questions:
Think about the friendships in your life that may be affecting your happiness.

Ask yourself: do you at times avoid these people? Maybe you screen their calls or you avoid doing the things you love because you know they will be there? Warning bells are ringing!

If you identify this as true, then it's time to create change.

Be the example.

Whether people realise it or not, by you being a wonderful example, they may want in. If they gossip, you don't.

Know your boundaries or at least create them and let them be known. For example, you might say: 'It doesn't make me feel good when we gossip, I'm not going to participate in it any more, just so you know.' If they don't respect your boundaries, they aren't respecting you.

Understand that such people won't back down easily. It doesn't mean you need to pick a fight, just stay firm in what you believe and be gentle in reminding them. You don't need to defend or make excuses for yourself. Be firm and name what you want, even if to yourself in your own mind.

Toxic people will be drawn to those who are empathetic, soft and kind. You may for this reason feel like you're being mean when you're naming what you want but stand firm. It's ok to stand up for what you want and, even though there may be some short-term discomfort, the long-term happiness is worth it.

You don't need to be unhappy for the sake of others' happiness. And while we all have friends who are down at times, those who are toxic really do need to go. You don't need that kind of juju draining your positivity.

CHAPTER 8

What's the deal, 'down there'?

'There is no wrong way
to have a body.'

HANNE BLAKE

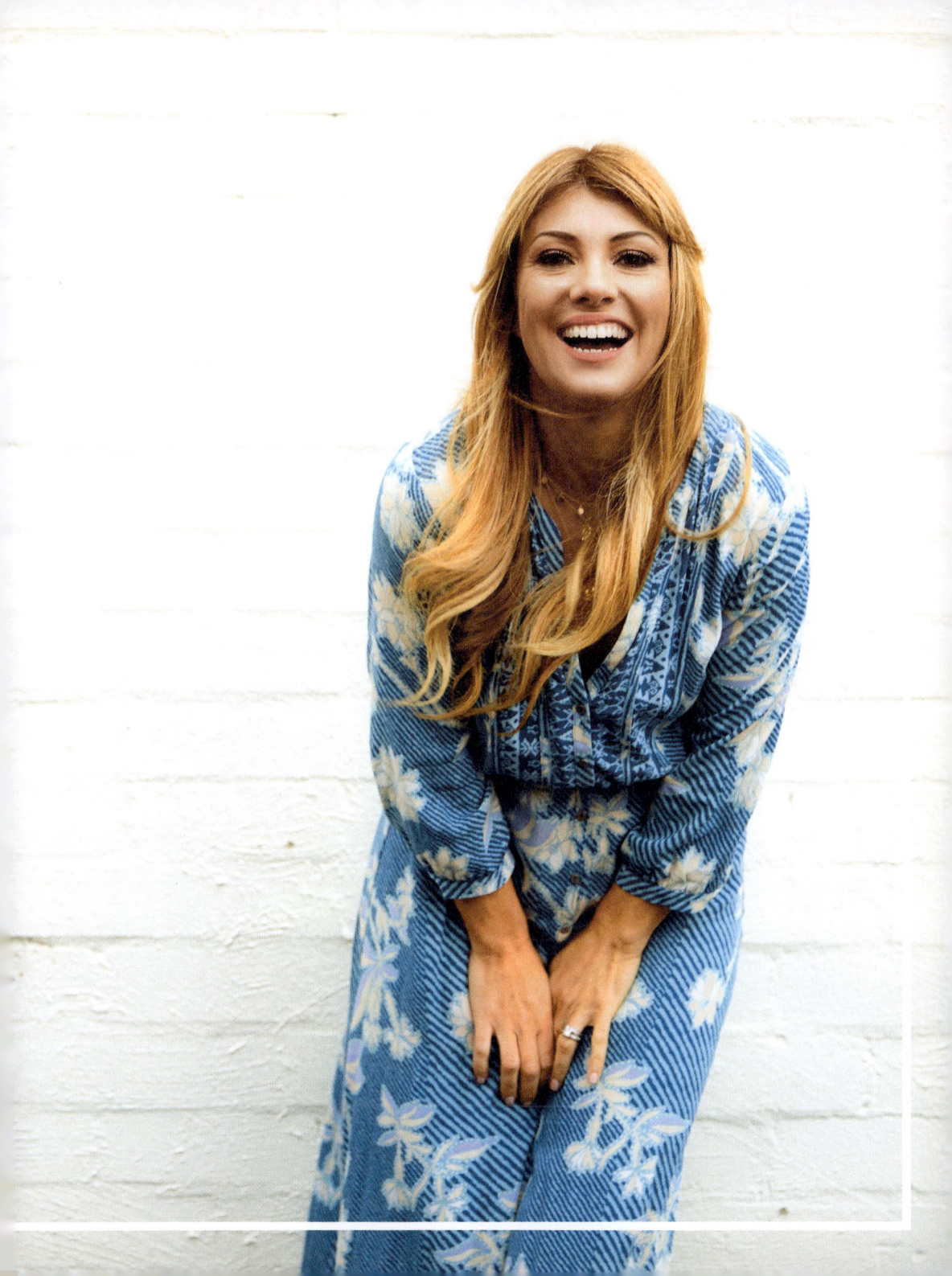

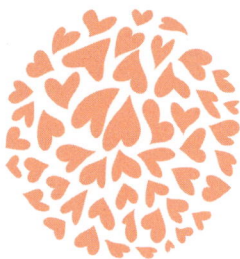

I swear that rogue hair wasn't there yesterday!

YOU WILL LEARN ABOUT:

• our anatomy • ovaries • fallopian tubes • uterus

• cervix • vagina • vulva • labia • urethra and bladder

• rectum • reproductive system • clitoris • orgasm

Really getting comfortable with your body and your anatomy I believe is where the game actually changes for us as women. I know as a young woman growing up my mother did a superior job in having the 'birds and the bees' talk. I had a book that I literally devoured, for weeks and weeks, possibly years on end. When I say book, it was an oversized pamphlet. It showed me cross sections of the uterus which resembled a deflated balloon and a few other squiggly lines, one representing the anus and the other the urethra. I don't remember there being much of a discussion about the cervix or the clitoris, or even the endometrial wall for that matter. Of course, it wasn't my mama's fault, she wasn't an artist or into line drawing and speaking of these areas of the body in detail was not so much taboo, but just not the done thing – being encouraged to 'tinker' about down there was certainly not part of the conversation. The booklet I had explained enough for me to learn the basic structure of my reproductive organs and explain my period. And the rest was up to my level of curiosity – a muscle which as young women we were typically not encouraged to use and so therefore I didn't.

Granted, I never got a mirror out down there to check things out, mostly because I was freaked out by it. I mean I waxed and made sure my pubic region didn't look like something from the 70s, but that was all for aesthetics; I never really knew much about what was what. I relied on the line drawings in my trusty pamphlet and assumed it looked something like what the drawings resembled. It really wasn't until I had children that I started to get curious about what things may have looked liked 'down there' and began to realise that no two vaginas are the same. Just like our nose or our teeth or our belly, we all look different. Probably the only one bonus in not talking about it was that as a teenager I wasn't comparing my vagina to my girlfriends', all because it just wasn't ever spoken about.

So let's take a look.

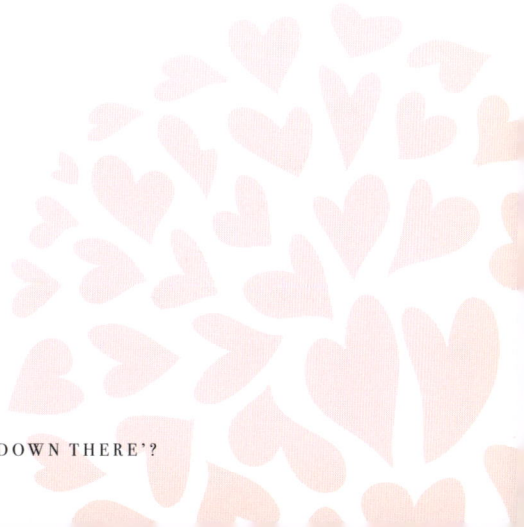

Our anatomy

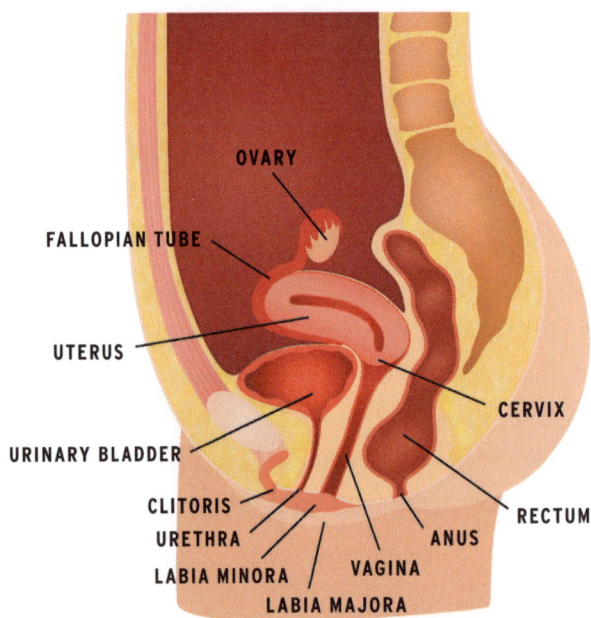

Diagram labels: OVARY, FALLOPIAN TUBE, UTERUS, URINARY BLADDER, CLITORIS, URETHRA, LABIA MINORA, LABIA MAJORA, VAGINA, ANUS, RECTUM, CERVIX

OVARIES

These are the olive-sized organs that house/produce the ova (eggs) each month. As well as this, they are endocrine glands because they secrete hormones, mostly oestrogen and progesterone (and later in life testosterone). The ova are what the sperm fertilise in conception, in which pregnancy results.

If you're curious about where your ovaries are, place both thumbs flat on your stomach with your thumbs in your belly. Join your index fingers to make a triangle shape – the index fingers being the point. Where your little fingers naturally sit are approximately where your ovaries lie. This can be useful if you experience pain in this area to pinpoint what is actually hurting.

FALLOPIAN TUBES

The tubes, known as the salpinges, provide an avenue for the egg to travel from the ovary to the uterus.

UTERUS

The top part of the uterus (the fundus) connects to the fallopian tube and the lower part opens to the cervix which leads into the vagina. It is the uterus that is also known as the womb, which is where an embryo implants into the lining (endometrium) and grows during pregnancy. It is the uterine lining or endometrium shedding each month which results in a period.

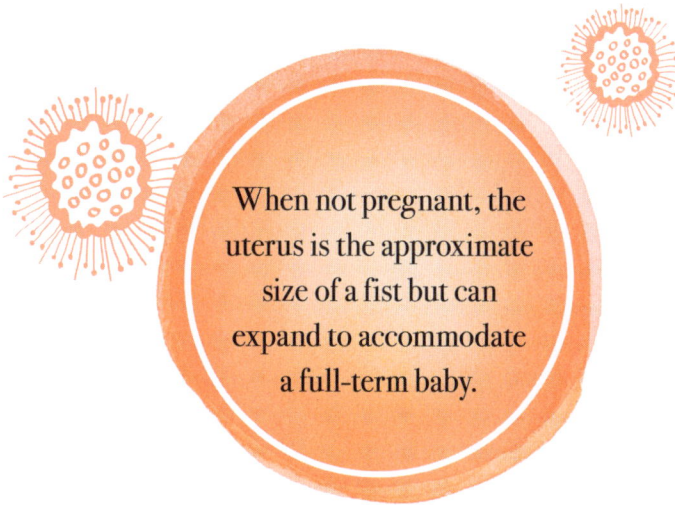

When not pregnant, the uterus is the approximate size of a fist but can expand to accommodate a full-term baby.

CERVIX

This is the lower part of the uterus, which connects to the vagina. The cervix is also where discharge or mucus is produced. Consider your cervix as the gatekeeper to your vagina. It opens during ovulation to let the sperm in and at various times of the cycle moves to accommodate what's going on with your body, hormonally. When looking at your cervix front on, it kind of resembles a donut. Here's a month of cervix activity:

- **Follicular phase** During this time, the cervix is high and closed.
- **Ovulation** The cervix moves down (in preparation to receive sperm in the act of conception). The cervix also opens to receive sperm should sex occur at this time.
- **Luteal phase** There's not much activity at this time so the cervix moves back up and is closed. The body is preparing for menstruation.
- **Menstruation** The cervix is open to allow the blood to leave the uterus and the period to flow.
- **During sex** An orgasm will see the cervix contract – an act that's thought to assist the sperm in moving through to the uterus. For some women, the sensation of the penis bumping the cervix may be pleasurable or may be uncomfortable. It really depends, because you guessed it, we're all different. (Keep reading – I've more on answering your questions if sex should be painful – the answer is no, FYI!)

Every cervix is different, which is why you might like to get familiar with your own unique self.

VAGINA

The vagina is the passage which connects the uterus to the external world of the body. It's full of nerve endings, which allow you to feel sensation. The most external part of the vagina is the vulva and the labia – they are the parts that you may be the most familiar with because you can see them.

VULVA

The vulva refers to the external sex organs including the pubis, labia, clitoris (more on this later, see page 203), the bulb of vestibule, vulva vestibule, the urinary meatus, the greater and lesser vestibular glands and the vaginal opening. We may confuse the vulva for the vagina but the vulva is external and connects to the vagina. You'll notice something – there is no such thing as a 'normal' vulva. Just like your fingerprints or your eye colour, we are all so different.

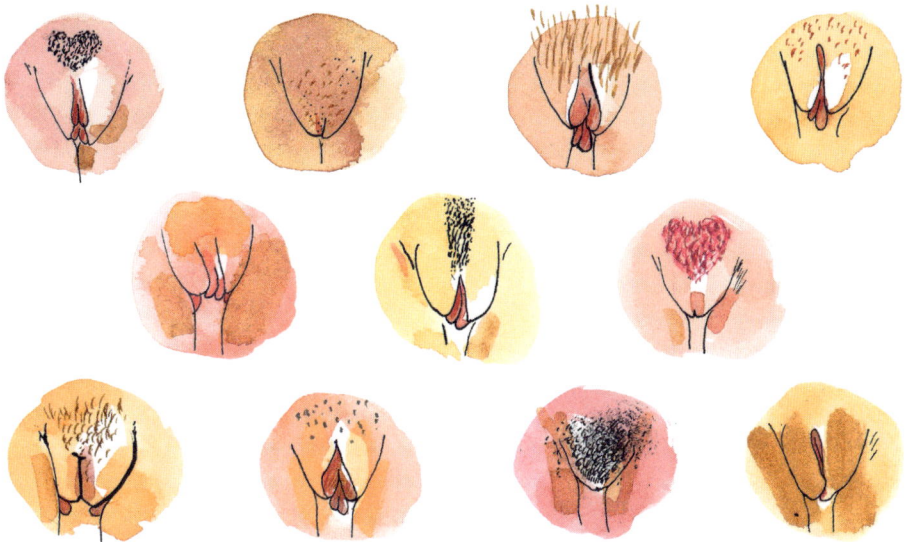

LABIA

Refers to the inner and outer folds, either side of the vagina. The labia minora are the more internal skin folds and the labia majora are the most outer. Remember, no two really look the same; some women's are smaller and some women's are larger. There's no right or wrong here. The purpose of the labia is to protect the vagina.

HYMEN

Before you are sexually active you will have a very thin membrane of tissue at the narrow part of the vaginal opening, known as the hymen. The hymen may be broken during sex or from exercise.

URETHRA AND BLADDER

The urethra connects to the bladder. You have three openings, the urethra where your urine is excreted, your vulva (as discussed), and your anus.

ANUS AND RECTUM

The last of the three orifices or openings, the anus is where you excrete fecal waste. The rectum is the section above the anus.

We're now going to talk about the reproductive system, sex and the clitoris.

REPRODUCTIVE SYSTEM

With so many important parts to your reproductive system, it's easy to get overwhelmed or ignore it altogether – after all, it's not like we can really see much of it and we're not always told much about it beyond its anatomic structure. I like to think the fact that our reproductive system is tucked out of sight isn't so much a design flaw, but rather serves an amazing purpose. Unlike males, who have more visible aspects to their reproductive system, our more internal counterpart is perfectly positioned. Nobody gets the short straw here really, when we think about it. For the boys, when it's time, their hormones really show up, they grow facial and body hair, their voice deepens and most embarrassingly at times, when they are aroused, it shows. They may also experience times when they're sleeping and ejaculate without any warning.

Personally, I'm beginning to feel privileged as a woman! We're a little more discreet in how things show up for us (thankfully), although sometimes our mood swings may make up for it. For us, the most apparent physical changes we see are when our breasts begin to grow. Thankfully, nobody knows when we have our period unless we tell them so – even though it might feel like everybody can tell, chances are unless you're publishing it, nobody else can tell at all.

After having my second child I definitely learnt this. My first born was a vaginal delivery and I didn't give too much thought to the fact that everything involved in the process of childbirth was completely out of the way, so to speak. It wasn't until the birth of my second child, who was a caesarean delivery, that I realised how perfectly positioned our most intimate parts are – completely out of harm's way and in the perfect position for recovery. Recovering from a c-section was much harder – everything involved with a baby, be it changing a nappy or feeding, saw to it that my wound was always in the firing line. But what's more, think about bleeding every month from any other part of your body: more than likely annoying and completely impossible for gravity to play its role if we were to bleed from any other place or area.

The only true way of us understanding anything better is to look further into it, yet the idea of deepening our understanding into our reproductive system weirdly comes with sexual association only. But our reproductive system isn't only sexual. We have specific hormones that are designed to be turned on for pleasure, but these aren't necessarily running frantic in our veins 24/7. In fact, quite the contrary.

Aside from pleasure, the role of the reproductive system is simply as the name suggests – for us to reproduce. This is the primary reason why we cycle each and every month, which can feel completely scary because falling pregnant this month may not be high on your to-do list and yet again, we're not taught that pregnancy can only happen when we are ovulating. **No egg (ovum), no conception, no baby. It's pretty simple and understanding your fertile times is one of the best gifts you can give yourself.**

It's totally normal to feel interested and curious about sex; in fact, part of the reason we may be so curious about it is because we don't really understand it properly and unfortunately there is no manual that comes with it, just like there is no real manual for birth or parenting – some of it has to be guided by what we innately feel. So given there's not a lot of information for us to tap into *and* unless we're sexually active, it's hard to have any idea of what's to be expected. Even though you may have seen people be intimate in the movies, truth be told, nothing really is like what you see on TV.

It's your body

Lucky for you, your body is yours and you get to learn about it to really show it who's boss. There are no rules with this, it's all about you, and you get to decide what to do when. But what is important is that we become confident enough to tap into what feels good for us in any given moment, which is going to be different for everybody. Just like no two labias are the same, no two bodies are the same either, which makes total sense.

I want to help you feel comfortable and safe enough to be curious, ask questions and learn about not only the parts of yourself that you can see, but also the parts that you can't. And if you're not at the point in your life where you're sexually active, even better – you're at the point in your life where you can feel free to explore your body to understand what's actually going on, what's what and what bit does what! Your body is 100% yours, so best to own it and understand it as much as possible. **Feeling comfortable and understanding** your own body first is the secret to being comfortable and relaxed when intimate. Give yourself a chance to understand this first before considering being intimate with anybody else.

Which brings me to your clitoris.

CLITORIS

I read this in an article and it resonated with me greatly, because it explained that the clitoris doesn't get a lot of airtime, upstaged as it is by the vagina. Which in turn is left in the dust by all the attention the penis gets. This just strengthens my point. The penis gets way more attention, I believe, because we've accepted that boys' sexuality is far more 'out there' for all to see. We joke about it, laugh about it and I know my parents' generation approached this area of health as 'boys will be boys' and sent them to their room to sort themselves out. But for girls, it's not common as a parent to say 'darling go grab a mirror and check out your clitoris for future reference'. This doesn't generally happen. Again because we associate it with sexual pleasure, the poor clitoris doesn't get a look in. It's just a part of your body that you're not encouraged to know anything about, until such time that it isn't so taboo to talk about any longer; however, we've missed the boat on understanding it and we're now faced with the fact that we really don't know much about ourselves at all.

I know as a young woman I still had no idea how it worked. It was definitely part of my anatomy and all I knew was that, under the right circumstances, could maybe become aroused. There was no mirror and definitely no way my hands were prying open my labia to investigate. **It's time for a change.**

The clitoris' sole purpose is to bring a woman pleasure. That's it. It's not a design flaw, it's not a hiccup or mistake, it's there for a good reason. It is also made up of the exact same materials as the penis, just assembled in a different way. It has a tonne of nerve endings (more than a penis actually), glands, a foreskin (known as the hood, making it sound like a mean machine), a shaft and erectile tissue, meaning when it is aroused, it swells much like a penis does. The clitoris, however, is only a quarter visible, unlike a penis which spends its life totally external to the body. But wait, there's more …

It's not only the clitorial head, hood and shaft, there is also the urethral sponge, the vestibular bulbs and the crus (also known as the clitoral legs - it's beginning to sound like a tadpole, I'd agree). The urethral sponge is an area of tissue found between the pubic bone and the vaginal wall. Just like the penis, during arousal this becomes flooded with blood, making it feel swollen which compresses the urethra which helps to prevent urination during sexual activity (genius). The vestibular bulbs are two elongated masses of tissue that sit either side of the vaginal opening and are related to the clitoris. During arousal the bulbs become filled with blood. It is during the act of orgasm that the blood is released. If there is no orgasm, the blood eventually leaves the bulbs after some time (a couple of hours). The crura (or collectively the crus) of the clitoris are two outer tissue structures that act in a similar way to the vestibular bulbs (they are right alongside them). That's a lot to take in, I know!

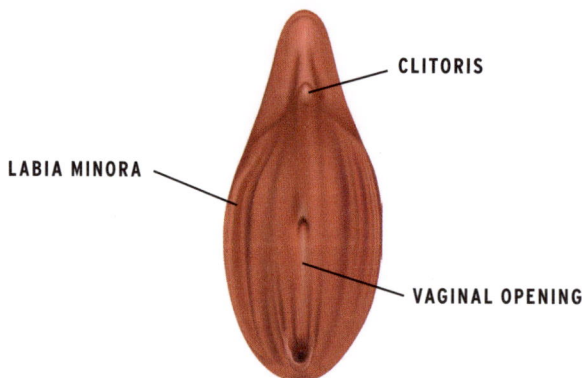

CLITORIS

LABIA MINORA

VAGINAL OPENING

Every bit of you
is part of you.

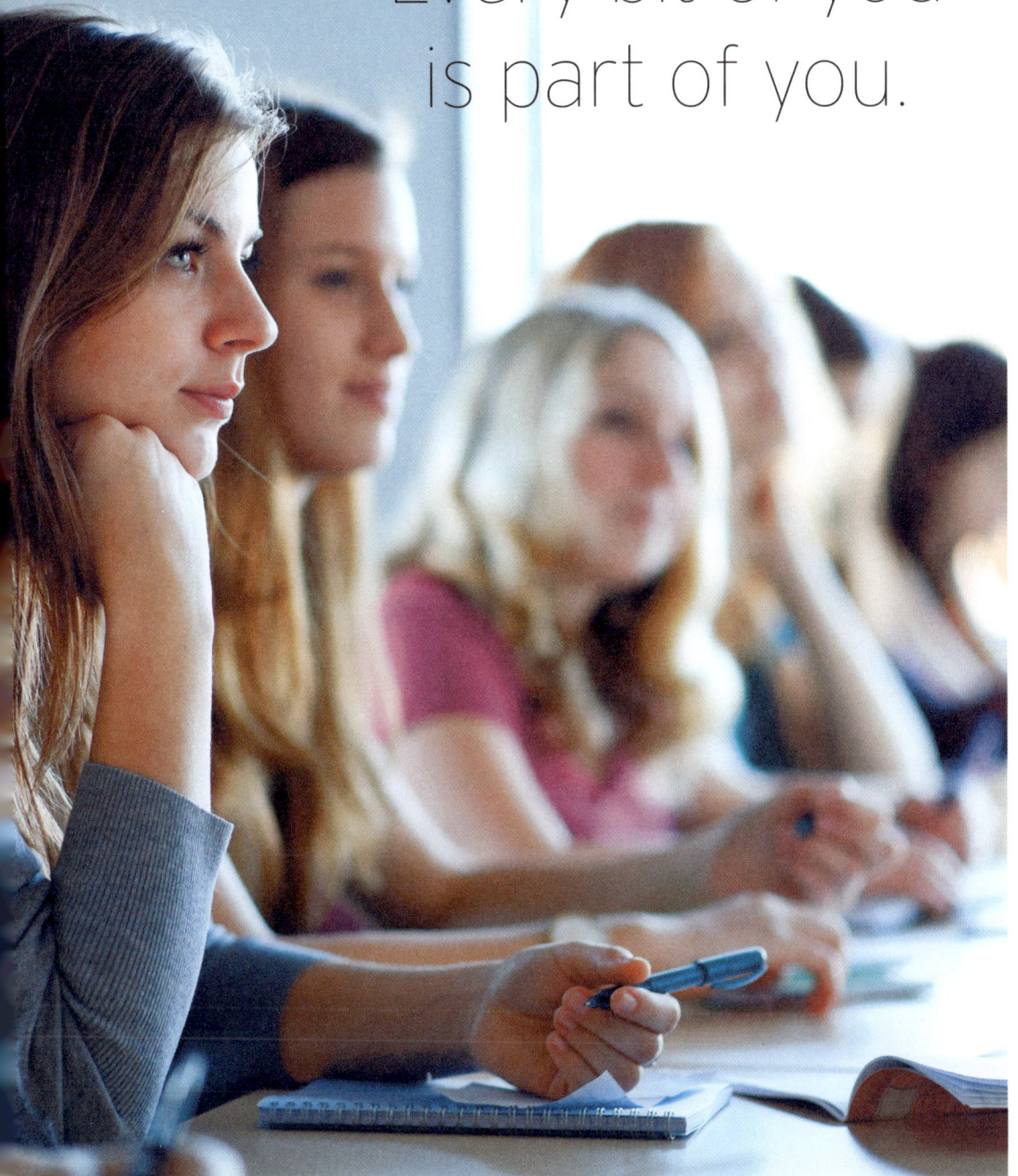

THE PUBIC REGION

It's not an anatomy lesson but more so a way of helping you make sense of all the 'pink bits' (the term may make you giggle but be reminded, we're all different and not all are pink!) you have, because let's face it there are so darn many. And because they all look so different, we can quickly begin to worry, especially if they look 'odd' (because let's face it, they naturally do look odd!), that there is something wrong, mostly because we've never taken the time to actually take a look at what we've got going on down there.

Now that you are well acquainted with your most intimate parts, it's important to understand that each and every part serves a very special purpose. The external parts of the pubic region are mostly related to protection and pleasure, while the more internal parts are related to procreation and preparation for an embryo, whether fertilisation occurs or not.

ORGASM

There are, of course, a few other areas that can become aroused and also lead to orgasm, just like the clitoris. Vaginal, cervical and G-spot orgasms can occur, although these are more difficult to achieve. In fact, it is said that up to 75% of women require clitoral stimulation for orgasm to occur.

You might wonder what actually is an orgasm?

First of all, not all women orgasm. Second of all, it can take a really long time to experience one – because when we become sexually active, we're learning about our bodies and what they are capable of. So let go of the idea that your first sexual encounter will be full of heat and passion. Probably not. You know, scientists still can't really figure out why we climax at all.

Basically what happens is during the act of sex, blood begins to rush to the clitoris, the cervix tightens and nerve and muscle tension builds until the body releases it all at once. That is what we know as an orgasm or climax.

Does everybody have orgasms? Nope, and not every time either.

Does an orgasm hurt? It shouldn't, although some areas can feel more sensitive to some than others and that's generally normal, too.

Can I have more than one orgasm? Yes, some women experience multiple orgasms.

Can I have an orgasm without having sex? Yes, by stimulating the clitoris (or any of the other sensitive areas mentioned) this can happen. Some women have reported sensations occurring during exercise or stretching.

The fact remains, an orgasm and feeling pleasure is a natural and normal part of being a human being. The most important thing you can do in relation to your body is understand your own anatomy and what happens, to allow you to explore this further and know it is ok to do so – just not maybe at the local bus stop but in the privacy of your bedroom or perhaps the shower. Don't be afraid of taking a look – it really isn't too different to checking out what's going on between your 4th and 5th toe or peeping up your nostril. It's all part of you!

So when should you have sex?

Like I mentioned, it is totally normal to feel interested or curious, but having sex just for the sake of it comes with a whole host of complications. There's a reason it isn't legal until 16 years of age – and we all mature differently. My advice – wait until it's something you feel comfortable with and with somebody you are totally relaxed with. You might wonder how you can feel completely comfortable, which most likely has nothing to do with the person you're being intimate with but more so exploring yourself so that you understand your body first. There is no perfect time for this and, while we may be told there are rules around what is best, the rules around understanding yourself haven't really been written – giving us permission to write these for ourselves. Having sex before you are of legal age can bring a whole host of complications and repercussions. In most places the age of consent is 16.

Many cultures and religions suggest that sex is a sacred event and I don't necessarily disagree. The act of sex itself is sacred and should be respected and happen in a nurturing environment. For me to stand here and tell you when that is for you isn't possible. But what I will say is the most important thing before having sex is ensuring that you have respect for yourself and a love for yourself.

Sex definitely creates a special bond between a couple. There are special hormones released during sex. Orgasm increases oestrogen and releases oxytocin.

DOES SEX HURT?

Well ... yes and no. The first time you have sex and lose your virginity, it will more than likely be a bit uncomfortable. You are going to be nervous and this can cause you to tighten your vaginal muscles (which are very strong, by the way). If you're nervous, you might be dry and lack lubrication (which is secreted in response to your feel-good hormones). This combination can cause some discomfort. If the sex is between a male and a female, let's also assume that young men have absolutely no experience and so might not have our pain in mind when the blood leaves their brains and goes to their penis. There can be other reasons later in life that sex is painful. For some women, it can be cultural or taboo to discuss sex and so they feel intimidated by sex and this combined with an unfamiliarity with their anatomy (see page 196 for my lovely anatomy lesson) can cause tension and pain. Other times, women might experience pain for reasons like endometriosis, adenomyosis, recent surgery in the area or just sometimes the muscles of the pelvis can be sore. Occasional pain, depending on the type of sexual positions, can be common and shouldn't cause alarm; you just need to educate your partner that things hurt a bit so they understand. If the pain is every time or most of the time, then you should visit a doctor who can do a proper examination. Now that we have that out of the way, sex is usually a wonderful thing and can be wonderful for you to bond with your partner. Mother Nature in all of her wisdom has made sex so enjoyable we want to keep doing it (thus continuing our existence on this planet). So, does sex hurt? Sometimes, but it shouldn't hurt all the time and mostly it should be a gift that you choose to share with a lucky person that you love who also understands the gift you are giving of yourself, and who should love and respect you equally. But please hear me when I say, the most important thing you can bring when being intimate is being comfortable with yourself first. This, I believe, is the key to making sex everything it is supposed to be.

CHAPTER 9

Your doctor

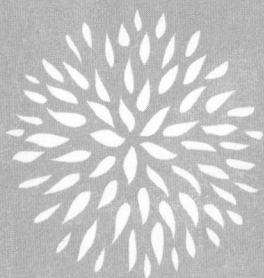

Nobody knows how you feel better than you.

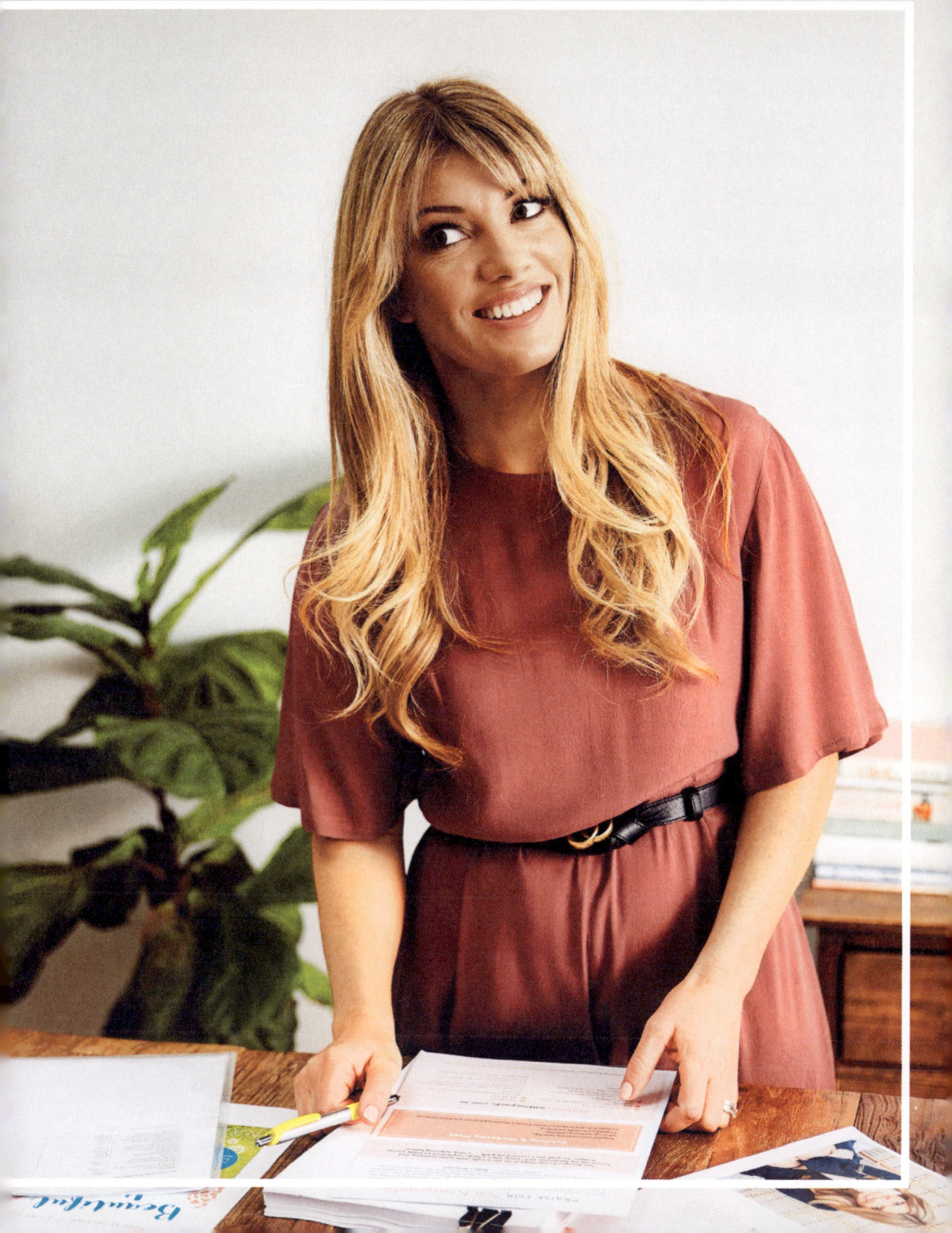

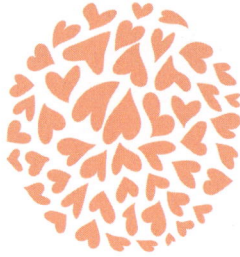

Only you know how you feel inside

YOU WILL LEARN ABOUT:

• frequently asked questions

This chapter is a collection of my most frequently asked questions. I had an overwhelming response on my social media channels when I asked what you wanted to know. (We should be friends there, by the way, so you can keep yourself updated and we can keep hanging out!)

WHY DO I GET SUCH BAD PERIOD PAIN AND OTHERS DON'T?

There are a few reasons. First up, lifestyle plays a huge role and this book is showing you how to make some fairly small changes to achieve some profound results. Try removing one of the following types of foods to see if there is a change. I recommend removing one for 21 days to see. Start with gluten and if your symptoms don't improve move onto dairy, and so on. Cold foods certainly congeal and stagnate blood flow. Try switching out cold and raw foods for warm and cooked foods. Caffeine has also been said to worsen period pain. It's a matter of trial and error to see what may work for you.

Remove one by one:

- Gluten
- Dairy
- Sugar
- Cold foods
- Caffeine

Will you always have period pain once you have it? Not if you do something about it. At the core of pain are lifestyle, diet and emotions. Diet is the easiest place to start. Your genetics and the state of your gut may be the deciding factor of your pain and where it decides to present for you.

> While you can't change your genes,
> you can manipulate your surroundings
> and your genes will follow your lead.

WILL I ALWAYS HAVE PERIOD PAIN?

Period pain has been accepted as being a normal monthly occurrence. I refer to period pain as a modern-day problem due to our current pace of life and general daily way of living. Good news is the more you fine-tune your body, the less niggles you'll experience. Period pain can be a thing of the past once you reduce things like stress and poor diet, which lead to inflammation and pain. See your doctor, however, if pain persists.

WHAT'S THE BEST DIET FOR PCOS?

The way you need to live for your body to thrive doesn't really change too much from person to person. Sure, some people are better with more protein and others with less but the fundamentals of what your hormones need to thrive doesn't change. Your hormones are made of fat and protein and for this reason, these foods should be abundant in your diet. (Good fats, I mean.) Foods that support healthy digestion are also key. Traditional Chinese Medicine subscribes to less cold and raw foods and more warm and cooked foods as an added layer to treatment and supporting your health. Tackle your PCOS and all hormone imbalance with a few key additions (and subtractions):

- reduce inflammatory foods (gluten, sugar and dairy)
- add ferments (probiotics) and collagen (found in slow-cooked meats, soups and stews)
- follow a wholefood diet, for most women with hormone imbalance a diet low in grains is best.

HOW DO I DEAL WITH OVULATION PAIN?

What I have found in clinic is that ovulation pain or pain in the middle of your menstrual cycle, typically around cycle day 13–15, is a sure sign of excess oestrogen. It is classic hormone imbalance, usually driven by stress of some kind. For young women, it's often worse during a period of heightened pressure, like exams or performances. I have patients during these times increase the amount of magnesium they are taking, just a little to see if it helps. I also advise that they ensure they have plenty of magnesium-rich foods, such as avocados, green leafy vegetables and bananas, in their diet at these times.

DOES IT MATTER IF I'M TAKING THE PILL? WHAT DOES IT DO LONG TERM?

The pill, like other hormone-based contraceptives such as Depo Provera injections, disrupts the natural state of your hormones – in fact, it flatlines them. The only benefit to the pill other than preventing unwanted pregnancy (which may be a big deal, I understand) is that you can cease taking it at any time, unlike the mirena, implants or an IUD, which need to be removed.

Sadly, the pill (including all synthetic hormone contraceptives) disrupts the health of the gut (the microbiome as well as the gut lining), it depletes essential vitamins and minerals and can come with a host of side effects, which commonly include changes in mood, headaches, low libido and blood clots. Taking the pill shouldn't be a decision made lightly – I always have patients ask themselves if it is treating a problem or a symptom. If it's the latter, then there's more than likely another way without the side effects. Long term, the pill and other hormone-based birth control methods may be linked to infertility and other hormone issues like amenorrhea and PCOS.

IF I HAVE INJECTIONS FOR BIRTH CONTROL, HOW LONG AFTER STOPPING CAN I FALL PREGNANT?

This question is tricky to answer because we may all have differing levels of health post-birth control. But as a general rule, I suggest patients use six months to get their body back on track, replenish vitamin and mineral stores and re-establish the menstrual cycle before trying to conceive. Plus, the unborn child inherits its mother's gut health – we want to make sure that's on track too!

IF I HAVE PCOS, AM I INFERTILE?

No. The trick is supporting your body in the right way with the right diet and lifestyle, and understanding your cycles. PCOS doesn't mean you are infertile at all. In fact, women with PCOS are the best at conceiving in a state of famine (not that this is likely but it is an interesting fact) due to the nature of PCOS. This may also be why losing as little as 2 kilograms in weight can really assist in managing PCOS.

IF I HAVE ENDOMETRIOSIS, WILL I HAVE TROUBLE CONCEIVING?

An embryo certainly does like to land in a healthy uterine lining and in the case of endometriosis, depending where it is located, it can be a bit of a disruption. I always encourage patients to put their best foot forward and begin to address these issues when they are first diagnosed so they are not a hurdle in long-term health. Plenty of women with endometriosis fall pregnant, but addressing endometriosis may make pregnancy easier.

WHAT IS THE WEIRD, STICKY STUFF I SEE IN MY UNDERWEAR? IS IT NORMAL?

Cervical mucus or discharge is very normal. You might notice that the amount changes from day to day and the consistency changes, too. Mucus that is white or clear indicates a healthy cervix. That which is green, really yellow or smelly may need to be investigated. Just another way your body is communicating with you each month. The cervix secretes this as part of a healthy, fertile body. Cervical mucus seen at ovulation time is generally different to what we see at the other times of the cycle; it's more wet and slippery. If you are to look at it under a microscope, you'd find it's a series of channels which actually act like a freeway to allow the sperm to reach the egg. Other mucus you see outside of this time looks very different, more like a matrix pattern and doesn't assist the sperm.

IS IT NORMAL FOR MY DISCHARGE TO SMELL?

Depends on the smell. It can often smell a little like bleach or a little acidic but when it becomes offensive and fishy ongoing, it's a good idea to have it checked out. Also think of when your last shower was or if you've been in a sweaty environment as this can contribute to it smelling badly. If it is a one off, don't worry, but if it extends over several days, see your doctor.

HOW MUCH DISCHARGE IS NORMAL?

Everybody is different so it's not really about how much there is that would ring alarm bells but rather if there are any other concerning characteristics like smell and colour. You'll also notice more discharge in your ovulation window, which is normal, and sometimes a little extra just before the period is due. Many women see a 'plug' made of mucus that comes away just before the period, too. This is normal; not all women see this but it's certainly nothing to worry about.

DOES CERVICAL MUCUS OR DISCHARGE MEAN I HAVE THRUSH?

Not when it is healthy. Be wary if it resembles cottage cheese and is accompanied with itching or burning. Thrush is typically characterised by these symptoms. The best option for thrush (aka candida) is addressing the flora, increasing probiotics and reducing foods such as sugar and gluten that will feed the issue. Consult your doctor if you have recurrent thrush.

CAN I GET PREGNANT AT ANY TIME?

I'm so glad to set this record straight. No. You can only fall pregnant when you're ovulating – the trick is understanding when that is, which is what we are going to begin to establish in the diary section of this book.

I don't want it to be hard for you to know when you are ovulating, and once you understand this, it may open up a whole new world to your body. However, because you may still find it confusing or you haven't been taught correctly, it may be hard to know when you're ovulating and because the period of ovulation may vary, it's wise to be very careful and either not have sex or use contraceptives if you do not want to get pregnant. We're working on that though – aren't we?

> If you don't know for sure when you're ovulating, it's wise to be very careful and either not have sex or use contraceptives if you do not want to get pregnant.

CAN I GET PREGNANT WITHOUT PENETRATION?

No. During the course of sex, the act of ejaculation propels the sperm into the cervix. From here, the sperm begin to make their way to the egg, but it doesn't happen at lightning speed. There also needs to be fertile mucus present which assists the sperm reaching the egg. There really is a sequence of events that occur for conception to take place.

WHY DID I GET PRESCRIBED THE PILL FOR MY ACNE?

This may be because the person prescribing it didn't realise there are many ways to achieve a result, or you were keen for a rapid result. The pill is the prescription of choice for many hormone imbalance issues because it literally shuts down your own hormones' ebbs and flows. This is wonderful in theory although, as we've learnt, the long-term use isn't so much about its direct effect on your hormones (this is secondary) but how it upsets the core of your health. The pill may be a wonderful short-term option, but long term, it can't fix the problems at hand. I'm all for long-term solutions.

HOW DOES THE PILL FIX MY OVARIAN CYSTS?

It doesn't technically fix them, it stops your hormones from 'cycling' each month. In the case of ovarian cysts or multiple follicles like we see in PCOS, it can stop the follicles from developing but the minute you stop taking the pill, chances are you're right back where you started. Again, this is a short-term 'fix' but not a long-term solution.

IS IT NORMAL TO BLEED A LOT WHILE ON THE PILL?

No it is not. I most commonly see this when a patient has been on the pill for some time and it's asking for you to look more into what is going on. Definitely a sign to investigate.

IF I DON'T WANT TO TAKE THE PILL, WHAT ARE MY OPTIONS?

It depends on what you are wanting to achieve. This book is teaching you how to understand your body and your peak fertile times, which can act as awareness to prevent pregnancy.

HOW EFFECTIVE IS FAM?

When practised correctly, this method is approximately somewhere between 76% and 91% effective. FAM stands for Fertility Awareness Method, another name coined for understanding your menstrual cycles just like I'm teaching you in this book. This is not to be confused with the rhythm method or the calendar method – these methods do not look at the individual but rather assume everybody has 28 day cycles. You can increase the effectiveness of FAM by investing in a fertility monitor, which can increase the effectiveness to be up to 99%. Not only is it an excellent option, I believe all women should understand their own body rhythms no matter what. It's important to understand that FAM takes time and discipline. It must be practised correctly and if you are at a stage in your life when you can't give this your full attention and use it properly, possibly other forms of contraception may be better for you.

WILL MY BODY EVER FEEL NORMAL?

If you give it the love and care it is begging for, yes of course. Remember this relies on internal, external and emotional health concerns being met. If you've ticked off all the physical boxes – you sleep enough, your diet is amazing, you move your body and care for yourself – it can often be the emotional aspect that is waiting to be sorted. But sometimes we can't do this without ticking these physical boxes. Remember, you are a work in progress and rather than attaching to the goal of 'perfect health', attach to the feeling of how this would make you feel, and use this to help you through the tricky times.

IS IT OK TO SKIP MY PERIOD ON THE PILL?

As we learnt in Chapter 1, the period serves great purpose. Skipping it isn't fabulous for various reasons, including the cleansing of the menses and keeping the vaginal environment healthy. If you skip your period for too long, the uterus lining may become too thick; you need to have a period. As a once off, I understand there are times women may want to use the pill to skip their period. Long term, I don't think it is a healthy choice – but that's just my opinion. Shawn Tassone, MD, states, 'It's good to have at least 3-4 periods a year to make sure the lining is being cleaned out.'

HOW MUCH PERIOD PAIN IS NORMAL?

None! Period pain doesn't have to be there. It is a very common modern-day symptom that tells you something is up – be it inflammation from average gut health right through to something more stubborn like endometriosis. It's the perfect symptom to prompt you to investigate.

SHOULD I BE WORRIED IF MY VAGINA ISN'T SYMMETRICAL?

Definitely not. Nobody is 100% symmetrical. Consider it your secret superpower ... why not?

CHAPTER 10

You are what you eat

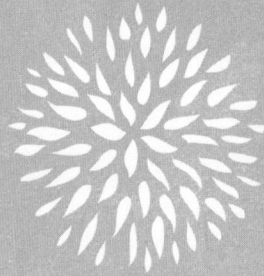

Change only one
thing - nutrition - and
watch your body thrive.

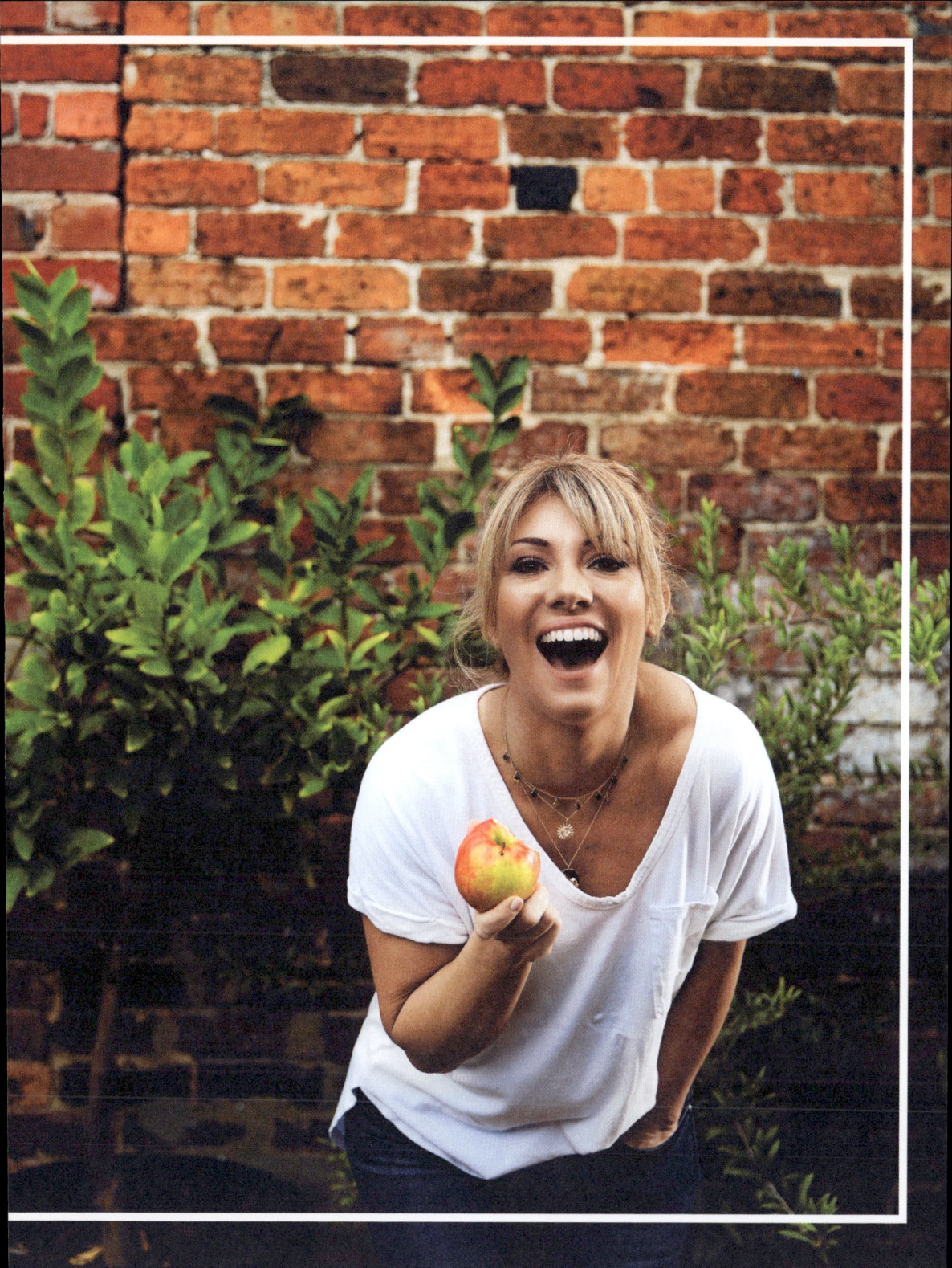

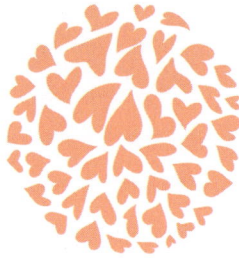

Nobody wants to be a hotdog

You've probably heard your granny say, 'you are what you eat!' and you've rolled your eyes mostly because you don't actually feel like a BLT sandwich. What does that even mean? But food is one of two things, remember? It is either of benefit or deficit to our body and it will undoubtedly take our health one of two directions – health or illness. There is no in-between. Can you get away with a few treats here and there? Please. Living it up a little is a must and you should be enjoying treats sporadically. But can you actually live on KFC? Well, as I learnt, it was only feeding my own poor health and hormone issues. These junk foods weren't able to be metabolised, offered little or no nutritional value and so often included foods that drove my insides crazy, leaving me nutritionally in deficit, and so I ended up also eating more because these foods were empty nutritionally.

So as the saying goes, 'you are what you eat'; if you are feasting out daily on donuts and hotdogs (that is, inflammatory foods), then you may well find yourself a ball of inflammation.

DITCH THE JUNK

It may be high time to ditch the junk – but before we jump into the overhaul, it may be more beneficial to start to focus on what you can include rather than what you should do away with. In one of my earlier books, I wrote, 'if you can pick it, pluck it or catch it, you should eat it'.

This leaves me asking you the question, when's the last time you saw a hotdog growing on a hotdog bush? Our modern world is chock-full of processed and refined foods and sadly much of their chemical ingredients are highly addictive, and unless you have yourself a degree in food science it can be so hard to know what all the ingredients, numbers and big words on the side of a packet mean.

There's an easy solution – wholefoods. These are those foods that grow in the ground, on trees or roam the land. We stick to these and we're off to a great start. Nature has it all worked out for us and truly, after all is said and done, I'm all about ease – let's work smarter, not harder.

'You are what you eat.'

So rather than feeling the guilts every time you grab a sneaky snack on the run, what if you simply asked yourself, is this snack helping me? Switch out a chocolate bar for a cleaner version of itself (the next chapter has some amazing recipes that you can very easily get yourself sorted).

I find that the biggest factor in changing your food habits is preparation. When we aren't prepared, it's easier to grab the unhealthy option. In fact, it's always going to be easier, but this is the commitment you're making to yourself and your long-term health – to be fabulous, glowing, healthy and feeling amazing, because you are worth that investment. No retail therapy can compare to feeling good.

GOOD FATS

The second secret I have for you in fueling your body for success is fat. When I was a young woman, I got scared out of eating fat because we were being fed bad science – that fat made us fat. But it couldn't be further from the truth and fat may well be your secret weapon to amazing health.

In the 80s and 90s it was fed to us that fat was leading to issues like heart disease, high cholesterol, heart attacks and so on. American scientist Ancel Keys observed that people who had a diet high in fat were more likely to develop heart disease, so he went on a crusade encouraging us all to cut the fat. His logic was that when you ate fat, this directly transferred to your heart, your arteries and around your organs.

But there was a fault in his research. Most of the cultures he observed in his studies had the same Western diet. Had he gathered information using varying cultural groups like Greeks or Inuits, he would have found that some cultures have extremely high fat consumption yet very low rates of heart disease.

His research was actually flawed, yet to date, many people don't realise that good fats are the secret weapon to health, youth and vitality. What's more, your hormones are made of fat and protein, so of course it makes total sense to make sure there is plenty of this in your diet to tick this box alone. But the benefits do not end there.

Good quality fats (those found in foods like nuts, seeds, oily fish, lean meats, avocados and eggs) help you to feel satisfied, help you to feel fuller for longer and help keep a healthy weight in check.

They interact with a part of our brain called the amygdala and tells us we've eaten enough. It's actually physically impossible to overeat good fats, your body simply won't allow you to - you stop because you feel content (satiated).

You'll be pleased to feel the relief when I tell you (good) fat is your friend. (Oh, but we're not talking about fast foods or highly fried foods because, remember, we left those well alone and are on the wholefood train now.) The fat you have circulating in your body is an essential energy source and vital life ingredient that we get from food.

Fat doesn't make us fat. Sugar on the other hand can be standing between you and your healthier self.

Your other best friend alongside fat is protein. My general rule is incorporating a fist size amount of protein at each meal alongside good fats and low GI carbohydrates.

I find the biggest issue for patients is having enough fat and protein at breakfast. But if you can get this right, your sugar levels will be far more balanced during the day, you'll have fewer cravings and you should find you're less tired mid afternoon. The best benefit is you'll also be less hungry, which means more time to do the things you love. Food becomes a wonderful part of your day, but not the focus of every waking thought because you are nutritionally satisfied – your body isn't screaming for more because you haven't met its needs. It's happy and you feel it, inside and out.

So fat helps to support our hormones, it turns off the hunger mechanism, allows us to feel fuller for longer and is a delicious inclusion into our lives. There's nothing not to love. Fat is also necessary to support your healthy nervous system (if our hormones are the messengers our body needs to perform tasks, our nervous system is the hard wiring). Fat is a sustainable food source that should be present at each and every meal. I find this one very simple and delicious inclusion you can easily add to your routine without much fuss.

Changing the way you eat can feel completely overwhelming and for some isolating. But I'm here to help. Let's focus on one thing at a time to really get the ball rolling AND because the next chapter is dedicated to what's on your plate, we've not only got answers but solutions too.

Of course, once you begin to eat this way, I know that you will begin to feel amazing, your sleep will become deeper, you'll be more productive, your brain sharper, you'll feel good in your skin and your weight will be healthy with fairly little effort. That's just the beginning, though; your pain-free periods are on their way, your clearer skin or pesky hormone issues may also be less of an issue, all from some little shifts. But treat it as an experiment. Here's how.

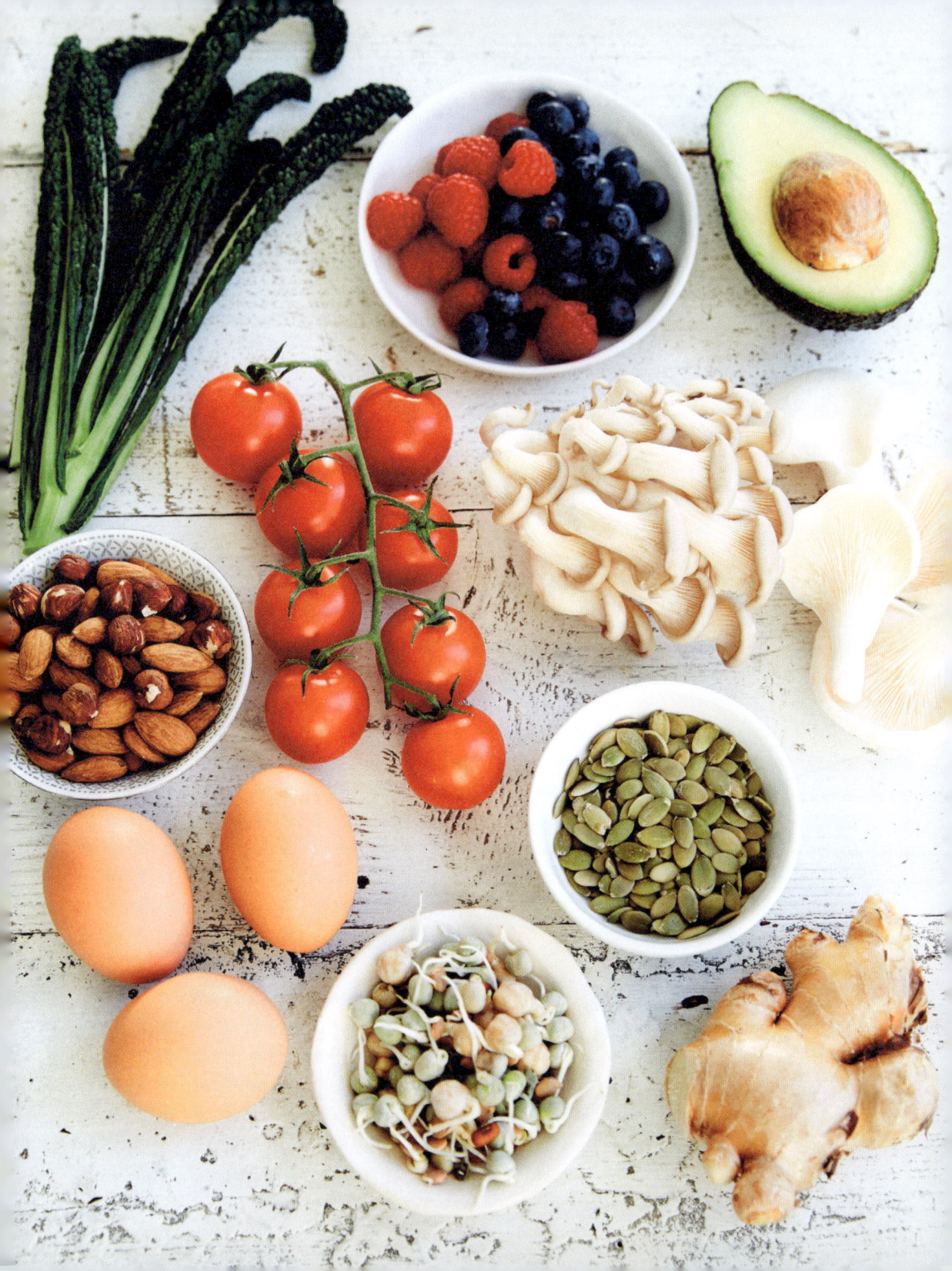

Getting on track with your food

For the next 4 weeks, we're going to help you get on track with your food. It starts with including the good foods first (and then if you're still hungry, eat what you'd normally eat).

WEEK 1

Add in good fats and protein to each meal, especially focusing on breakfast. These might include avocado, nuts, seeds, oily fish, eggs.

WEEK 2

It's time to cut the refined sugar. You've now acquainted yourself with some of the delicious snacks and fuel in the next chapter.

WEEK 3

If you have a known hormone imbalance like PCOS, it's time to lessen the dairy. We're told we need the calcium from milk, but sadly, we don't really get as much as we are led to believe, mostly due to the denaturation of milk in the pasteurisation process. For women with PCOS, dairy can be a disaster (you're consuming hormone-fuelled milk from a pregnant or postpartum cow) as it further disrupts hormones. Remember, it's just an experiment.

WEEK 4

Say goodbye to wheat gluten, just for the week, and check in with how your body feels. Switch to other ancient grains like spelt that, while still contain gluten, are far easier to digest.

During the 4 weeks it's a great time to introduce some fermented foods to the diet, like kombucha or fermented vegetables. These will help to replenish vital gut bacteria that life may have had its way with (allowing for overgrowth of the not so useful bacteria, the same ones that might be standing between you and your pain free self), as well as to increase gelatin and collagen to really support good gut integrity.

Remember you want the junctions of the cells of the gut wall to be strong and prevent any leakage that may be contributing to your inflammation and hormone imbalance. It's all a simple experiment to help drill down on your health and really get dialled into what works for you best. Your hormones will love you for it. **BUT EAT UP!**

Just because there are a few favourites on your list of foods that you normally eat that you are going to momentarily put to the side, you have a smorgasbord of food that awaits you. Consuming wholefoods is simple (we told you so) and delicious.

NOT SO PHAT

There are some stand-out fats that you should definitely avoid. These are typically hydrogenated or partly hydrogenated oils, oil blend margarines, canola, corn, vegetable, soybean, grapeseed, sunflower, safflower and rice bran oils, all of which are highly processed and pretty darn terrible for your insides.

You'll notice in the following chapter that the recipes tick the boxes in supporting you in your 4-week 'experiment'. I've ditched the flour by excluding bread and included recipes that don't contain gluten. What's more, gluten can play havoc with your hormones as it is converted to sugar and also causes the adrenals to become overworked due to the constant reaction to inflammation – it's not ideal, which may keep you in a constant state of hormone imbalance.

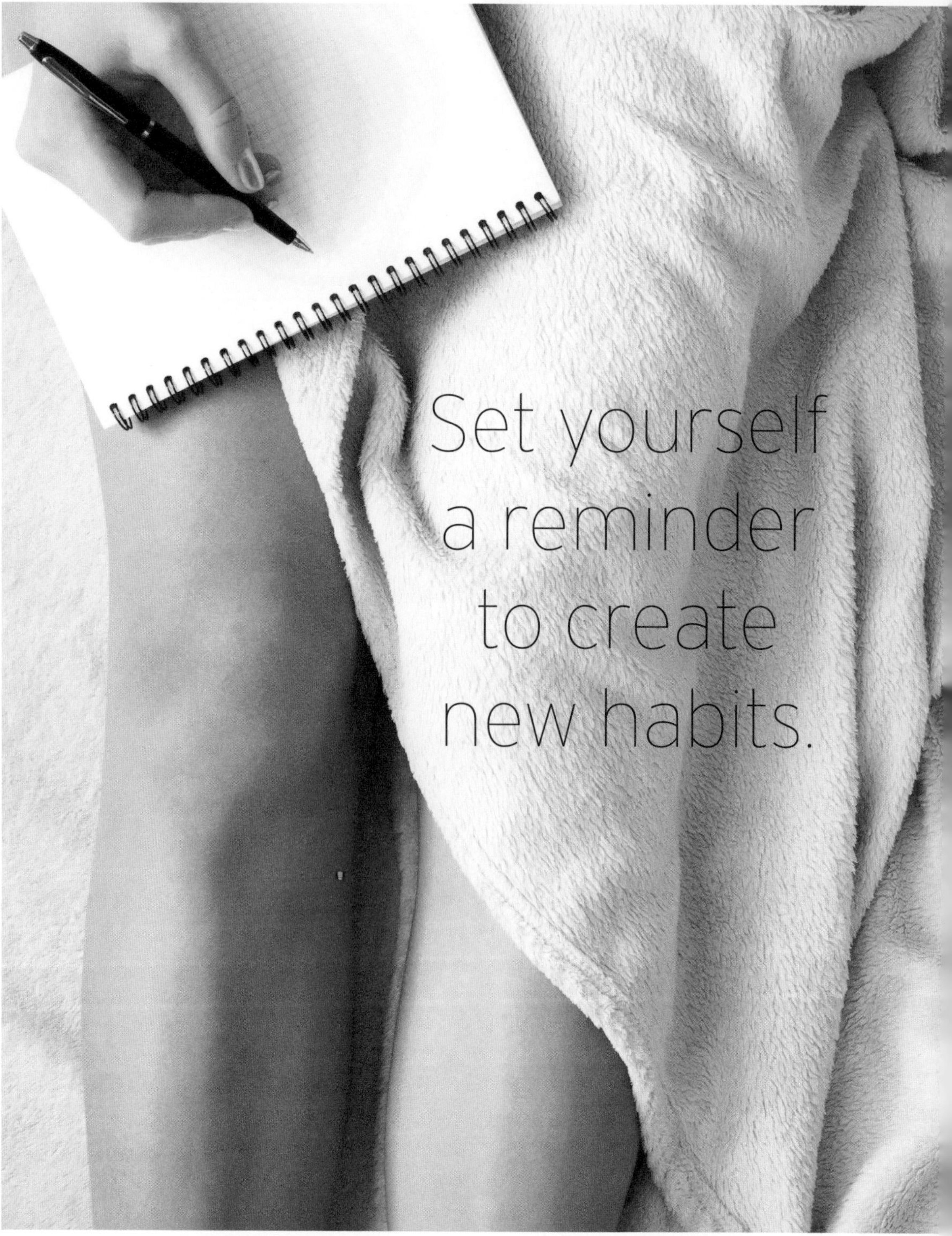

Set yourself
a reminder
to create
new habits.

Clean habits

It doesn't take too long to create a new habit. But as easily as we create it, we can fall out of habits that we once loved, too (sometimes this might work in your favour if you have a bad habit!). Some researchers suggest 21 days to form a new way, others say less. Maybe it comes down to the individual (since we're all different, this makes the most amount of sense to me). But as a general rule, there's one rule you need to follow to create a new habit: **JUST DO IT.**

Each day, set yourself a reminder in your phone or pin a sticky note to your forehead – whatever you need to do to remind yourself – but when it comes to creating new habits and goals around your food habits, you'll begin to feel so good, you'll wonder why you waited so long to start. The bottom line is, do it until it is a habit, be it a week or 21 days. Chances are once you've got to the 21-day mark, you'll know you've got this.

These habits don't just extend to food but your lifestyle, too. Here are a few other very important factors to consider that we talked through earlier:

- Stress
- Sleep hygiene
- Food planning
- Exercise scheduling
- See Chapter 4 for beating the bloat.

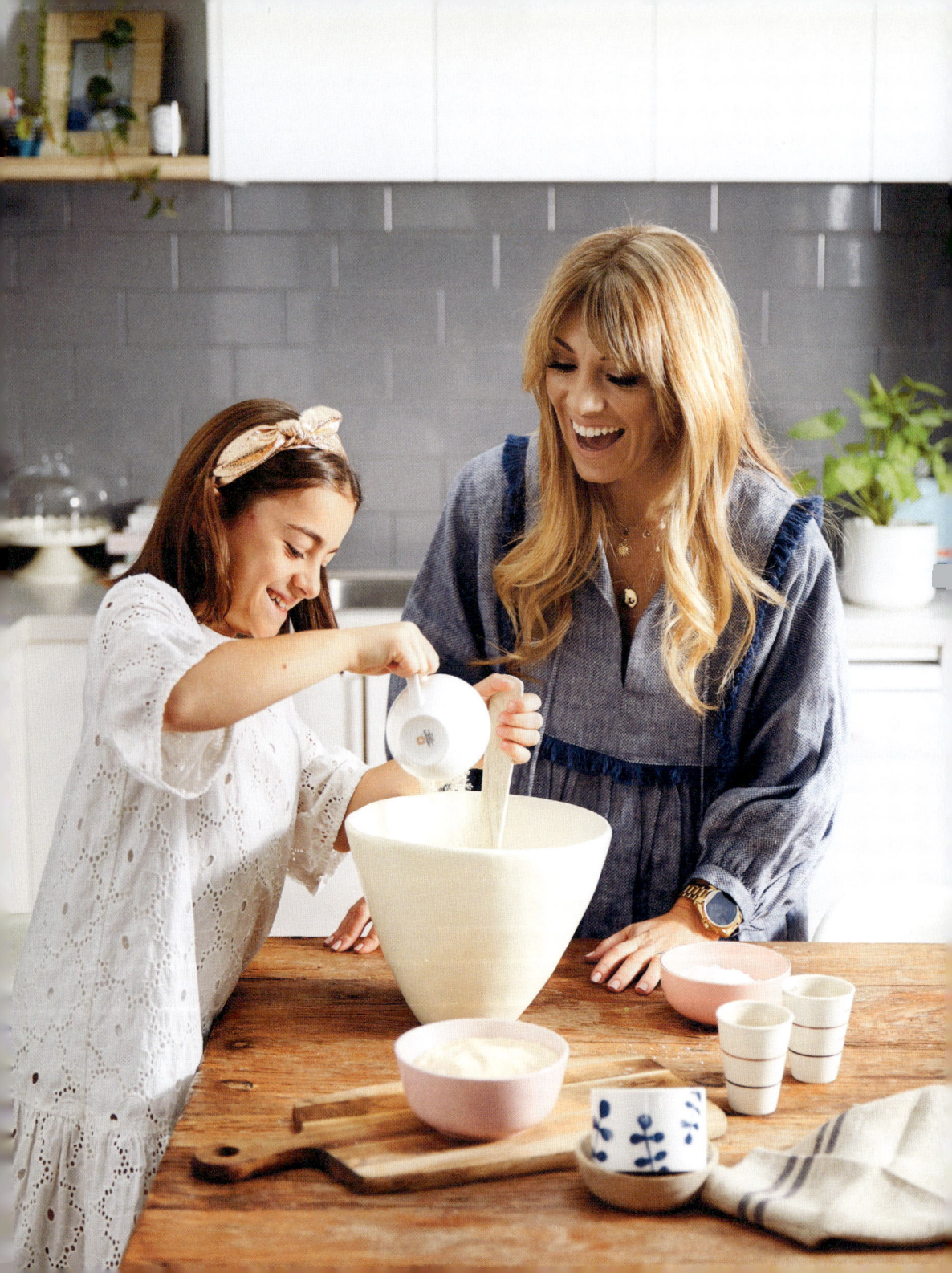

Your healthy and happy stomach

THE EPICENTRE OF YOUR HEALTH

It's so good that you now understand that food is indeed the foundation to your more hormonally balanced self – but without recipes to put this into practice, I feel that would be similar to baking you a cake and eating it in front of you. Unfair! So I've compiled some very quick, easy and delicious recipes that tick all the boxes – everything your hormones need from gluten-free chia puddings and pancakes, high-protein lunch bowls right through to fabulous snacks and treats that tick the boxes when it comes to fibre. All put together with your hormones in mind.

You'll find that the recipes are mostly free of gluten, dairy and refined sugar. You'll also notice that many serve just one. This is so you spend the time and make it for yourself – you can, of course, double or triple the recipes to suit.

Breakfast

I always encourage my patients to make breakfast count most. Breakfast may either make or break our insulin levels – you'll find these recipes tick the boxes of fat and protein to ensure your blood sugar is happy and your taste buds are equally satisfied

BREKKY BOWL

Brekky bowls are versatile and allow you to combine whatever healthy ingredients you like. They are a great option to prepare the evening before and grab on your way out the door.

1 handful berries, such as blueberries or raspberries

½ teaspoon honey

½ avocado

FOR TOPPING

1 banana, sliced

3 strawberries, sliced

1 handful nuts of your choice

1 teaspoon chia seeds

1. Combine berries, honey and avocado in a blender and blend until smooth and pour into a bowl, or simply mash them in a bowl with a fork.

2. Top with banana, strawberries, chia seeds and nuts or the toppings of your choice.

SERVES 1

CHOC BERRY CHIA PUDDING

Chia seeds are a wonderfully versatile food. They work well as an egg replacement and are packed full of protein, too. Prepare the night before, then top with berries and nuts for a morning treat.

3 tablespoons chia seeds

1 tablespoon protein powder (if protein powder isn't sweetened, add 1 tablespoon rice malt syrup or raw honey)

1 tablespoon peanut butter

½ tablespoon cacao

½ 95 g (3 oz) can coconut cream

1 handful berries, such as strawberries, raspberries or blueberries

1 tablespoon chopped nuts (optional)

SERVES 1

1. Combine chia seeds, protein powder, peanut butter, cacao and coconut cream in a glass bowl and stir well. The consistency will quickly become paste-like. Cover or transfer to a glass jar.

2. Place in refrigerator for 20-30 minutes or overnight to allow the chia to swell.

3. Top with berries and nuts.

ALMOST OMELETTE

I call this almost omelette because I'm terrible at making omelettes!
They always fall apart and I end up mixing it in the pan. Here's to
removing the pressure of becoming a masterchef!

2 tablespoons oil, for
frying

3 spring onions, sliced

5 mushrooms, chopped

5 cherry tomatoes,
halved

1 large handful spinach
leaves

2 organic free-range
eggs

salt and pepper, to taste

SERVES 1

1. Heat oil in a frying pan over medium heat, then
   add onions and stir for 30 seconds before adding
   mushrooms, tomatoes and spinach.

2. Using a spatula or wooden spoon, arrange
   ingredients so you can crack the two eggs on top
   of the vegetables. Crack eggs on top and cover
   with a saucepan lid.

3. Turn heat back and allow to cook for 3-5 minutes
   or until the yolks are cooked to your liking. Serve
   immediately, season with salt and pepper and enjoy.

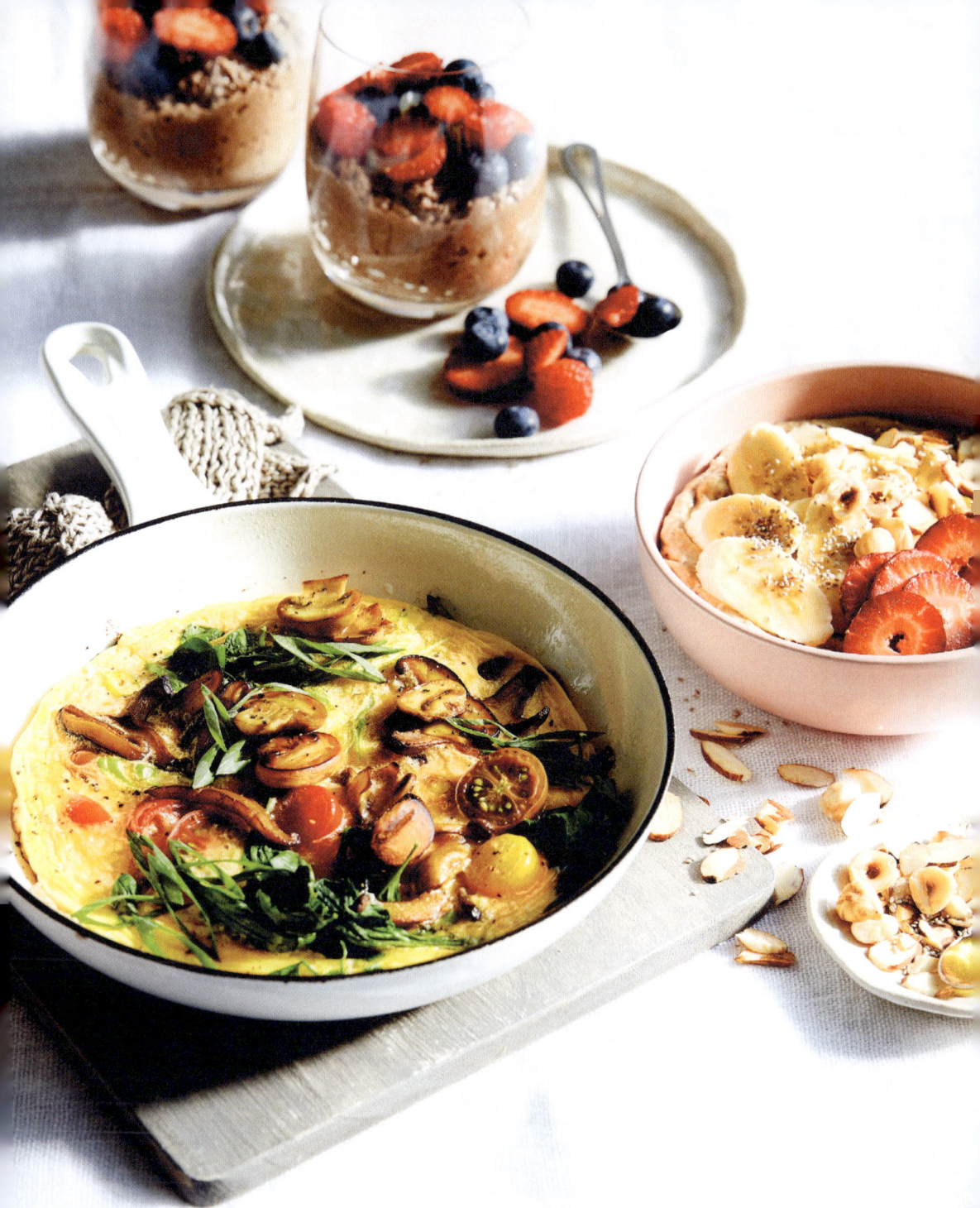

SWEET STRAWBERRY PARFAIT

This brekky parfait is made by layering warm chia jam with natural yoghurt.

2 cups strawberries,
chopped, plus extra
to serve

2 cups water

3 tablespoons honey

¼ cup chia seeds

1 cup plain natural yogurt

SERVES 1

1. To make chia jam, place chopped strawberries in a medium saucepan, add 2 cups of water to cover, and simmer over low heat until it begins to resemble jam. Stir occasionally and make sure it doesn't boil dry.

2. Add honey and mix well.

3. Add chia seeds and allow chia to swell and take on all the liquid.

4. Layer this in a tall glass with yoghurt and top with strawberries.

BANANA FRITTER CAKES

This is the simplest and quickest recipe you'll find. You can make
your own variation, using various fruits, nuts and seeds.

1 banana

1 egg

oil, for frying

1 handful raspberries
or blueberries

pure maple syrup,
if desired

SERVES 1

1. Mash the banana in a bowl. Beat the egg in another bowl.

2. Combine the egg and banana until well mixed.

3. Heat oil in a frying pan over medium heat. Pour batter
into frying pan and add berries. Flip when ready.

4. Serve immediately; drizzle with maple syrup if wanted.

BUCKWHEAT BERRY PANCAKES

These are an absolute favourite in my office. We've been known to cook up a batch before work and enjoy eating them together around the kitchen table. Seriously delicious and with the inclusion of buckwheat flour, these pancakes are gluten free!

1 cup buckwheat flour

½ cup rice milk

1 handful blueberries

coconut oil, for frying

SERVES 1-2

1. Combine ingredients in a bowl and use a whisk to beat until batter consistency (you may need to add more milk).

2. Heat coconut oil in a frying pan over medium heat. Pour the batter into the pan.

3. Garnish with the topping of your choice. Chia jam (see sweet strawberry parfait), berries, coconut yoghurt and honey are all great options.

Lunch

Most of these super easy lunch recipes can be prepared the night before, not only saving you time but ensuring you're doing your very best to look after your gut health and hormones throughout the day.

YUMMO CHICKEN SALAD

This can be as easy as having leftover chicken or a barbecue chicken (organic where possible or at least free range) in the fridge at the ready.

1 handful rocket or lettuce

3 strawberries, chopped

2 spring onions, chopped

½ avocado

1 cup chicken pulled from bone

1 tablespoon pine nuts

2 teaspoons apple cider vinegar

4 teaspoons extra virgin olive oil

salt and pepper, to taste

1. Combine rocket, berries, onion and avocado in a bowl or container.

2. Top with chicken and pine nuts.

3. Mix vinegar and oil, salt and pepper.

4. When ready to eat, add dressing.

SERVES 1

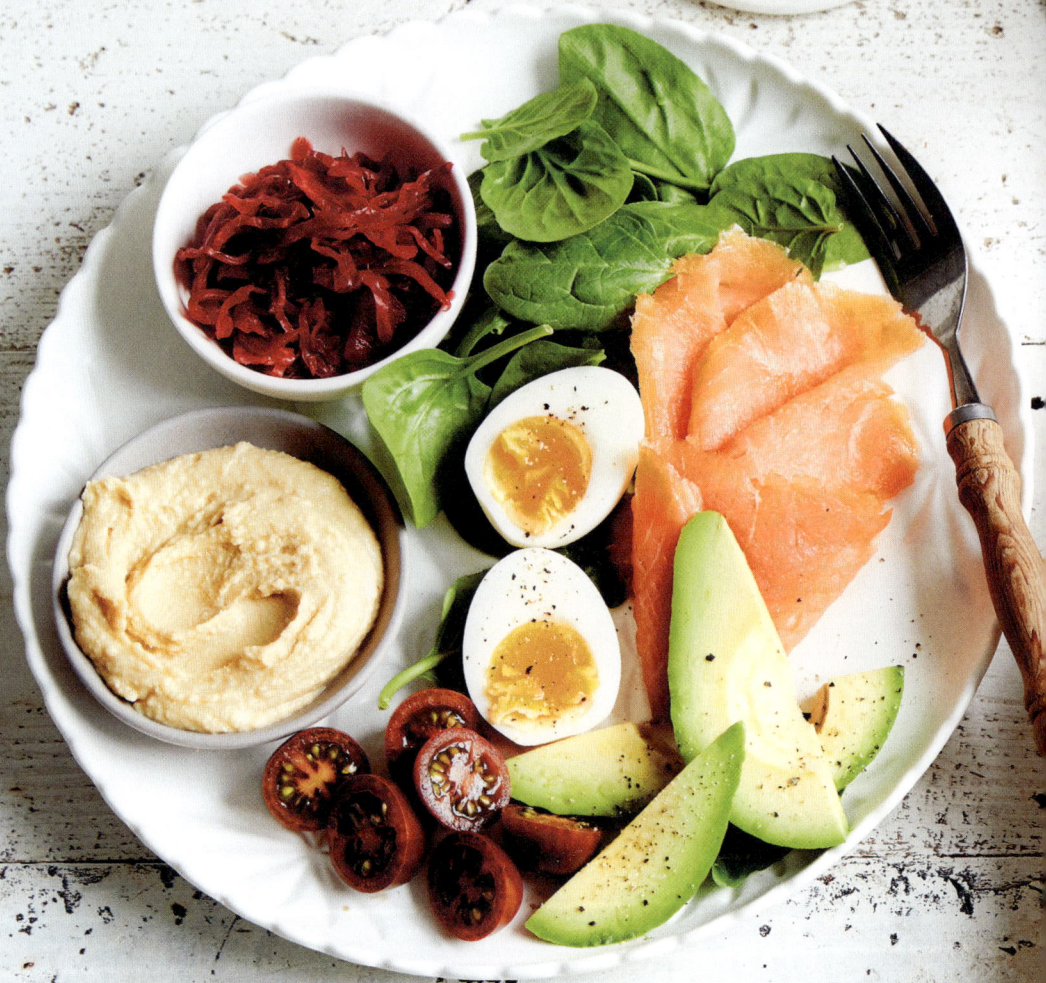

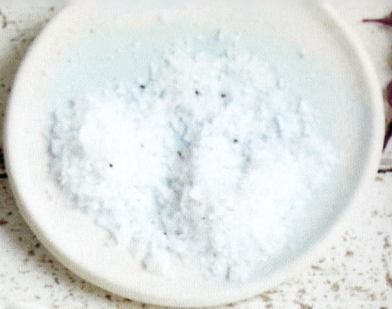

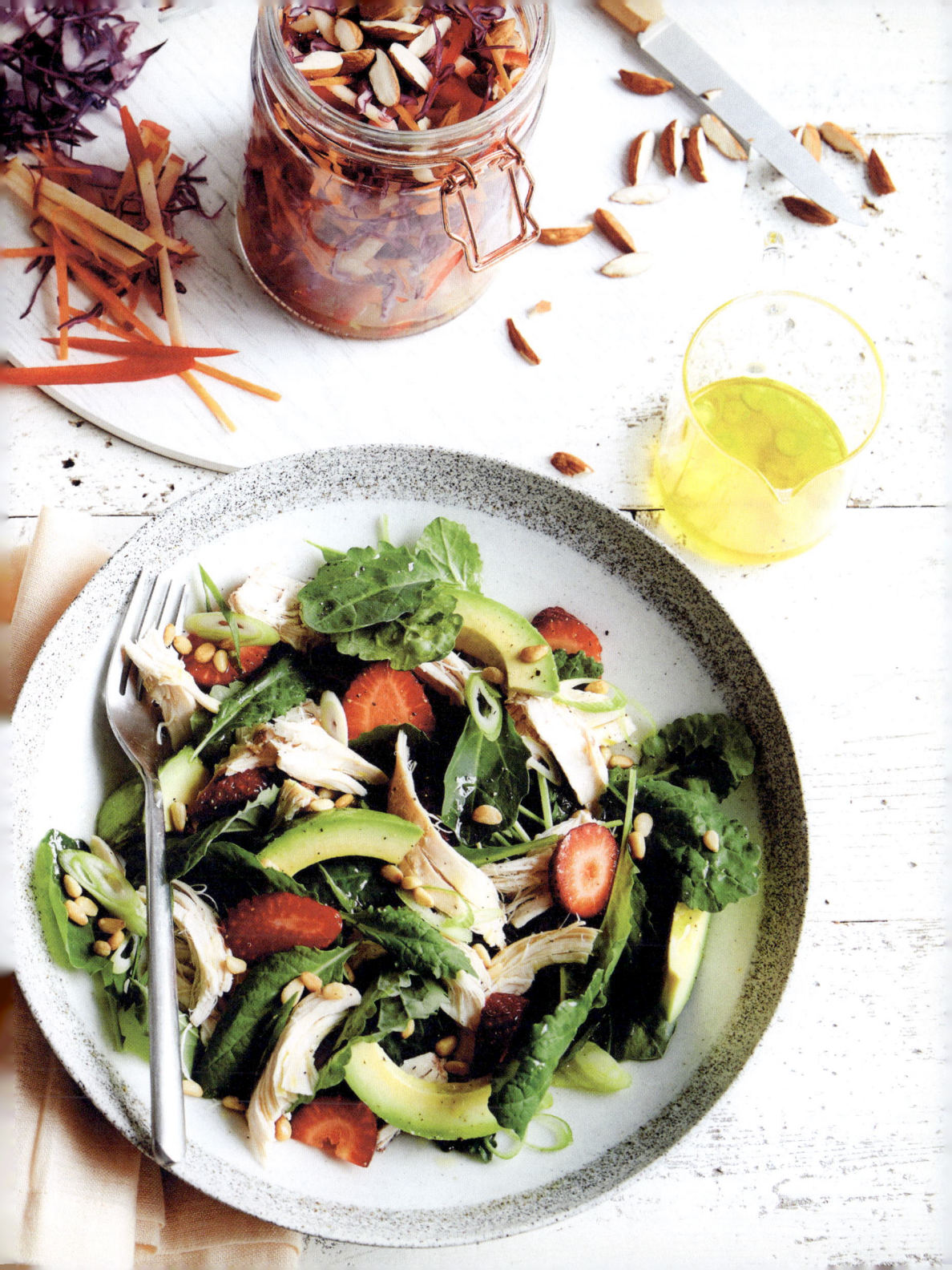

MISH-MASH LUNCH PLATE

There isn't necessarily a rhyme or reason to this recipe, simply use whatever you can find in the fridge. For me this changes daily and it may be a combo of leftover meat and/or vegetables plus some delicious additions like the ones I've included here. You can mix and match whatever you like.

Ideas to choose from and combine include:

boiled egg

spinach

grated carrot

grated apple

spiralised zucchini

1 can tuna

smoked salmon

fermented vegetables

avocado

olives

cherry tomatoes

hummus

bean shoots

nuts and seeds

SERVES 1

Mix and match whatever works for you – there's always something you can throw together if you keep healthy foods in your fridge and pantry.

SALAD JAR

This is so fun to make! It's literally making salad backwards by pouring the dressing into the bottom and allowing it to sit until ready to serve – when you're ready to eat, you shake the jar and allow the magic to happen!

1 cup finely sliced red cabbage

1 red capsicum, finely chopped

1 carrot, grated

1 apple, grated

5 almonds, chopped

DRESSING

2 tablespoons olive oil

2 tablespoons apple cider vinegar

1 clove garlic or 1 spring onion, chopped (optional)

salt and pepper, to taste

SERVES 1

1. Combine the vegetables and nuts in a small bowl and mix well.

2. Pour dressing into the bottom of the jar.

3. Top with vegetables – do not mix.

4. When ready to eat, turn the jar several times so dressing makes its way through the entire salad.

YOU ARE WHAT YOU EAT

SUSHI BOWL

You'll need either leftover chicken or a can of tuna for this recipe.

1 cup cooked rice of
your choice

½ cup cooked chicken
or canned tuna or any
protein of your choice

¼ cup cucumber,
chopped

1 sheet of nori, sliced

1 spring onion, chopped

1 teaspoon sesame seeds
(toasted even better)

seaweed salt, to sprinkle

SERVES 1

1. Arrange rice at the bottom of a bowl.

2. Place protein, cucumber and nori on top of the rice.

3. Top with spring onion and sesame seeds, and sprinkle
with seaweed salt.

TWISTED ZUCCHINI LUNCH BOWL

If you don't have a spiral vegetable cutter, cut the zucchini into thin slices with a knife. It won't be twisted but it will taste as good.

1 zucchini, spiralised

1 carrot, grated

1 cucumber, chopped

1 spring onion, sliced

195 g (3 oz) can tuna in olive oil

SERVES 1

1. Arrange ingredients in a container with the exception of the tuna.

2. When ready to eat, add tuna and enjoy.

LETTUCE CUPS

I like to have all the ingredients for this prepared in small containers and assemble when I'm ready to eat. Easy to pack and eat on the run.

95 g (3 oz) can quality tuna in oil

2-3 lettuce leaves (depending on how hungry you are!)

1 small carrot, grated

¼ thinly sliced or chopped capsicum

½ avocado, sliced when ready to eat

salt and pepper, to taste

SERVES 1

1. To make the 'cups', pull lettuce leaves from the head of an iceberg or butter lettuce.

2. Drain tuna and arrange tuna in each cup.

3. Top with carrot, capsicum and avocado.

4. Season with salt and pepper as desired.

Note: It's best not to cut the avocado until just before eating - it will turn brown from the air.

ANYTIME FRITTATA

You can experiment with this and add anything to the filling your heart so desires. This recipe calls for 500 g ricotta (which is delicious by the way) but if you are avoiding dairy, skip it or replace it with ½ cup almond milk and extra vegetables such as capsicum, or add in a can of tuna to really switch things up!

BASE

2 cups cooked brown rice

2 tablespoons butter (or coconut butter), melted

2 egg yolks (reserve whites for filling)

FILLING

500 g (16 oz) ricotta

2 eggs (plus whites from base)

4 spring onions, chopped

salt and pepper, to taste

2 bunches spinach or 1 bunch silverbeet, chopped

SERVES 6

1. Preheat oven to 200°C (395°F).

2. To make the base, mix rice and butter and fold through yolks in a medium bowl.

3. Grease a pie dish and press in the rice base firmly. Bake in oven for around 15 minutes or until it begins to brown.

4. Meanwhile, make the filling. If using ricotta, place in a bowl and mash with a potato masher until soft. Add eggs (and reserved whites), spring onion, salt and pepper and combine.

5. Fold through chopped spinach with ricotta or ricotta substitute to combine. Scoop onto rice base and bake for a further 20 minutes, or until top begins to brown.

Snacks and treats

We can find ourselves making a dash for the vending machine come 3 pm. The trick to avoiding that is having delicious healthy snacks at the ready! Here you'll find a variety of recipes, from cakes full of goodness that you can eat for breakfast right through to a personal favourite - bliss balls!

CHOCOLATE MOUSSE

Many years ago, I improvised this recipe when we had a dinner party - it turned out SO delicious I actually surprised myself! Cacao is a great source of magnesium and, let's face it, who doesn't love chocolate?

200 ml (7 oz) coconut cream

250 g (8 oz) dark chocolate, melted, plus extra to serve

2 teaspoons pure maple syrup

1 teaspoon peanut butter

SERVES 4

1. In a blender or mixer, combine all ingredients except extra chocolate, and mix until just smooth, without over mixing.

2. Pour into small dishes or glasses. Refrigerate for at least 2 hours.

3. Grate extra chocolate and sprinkle over to serve.

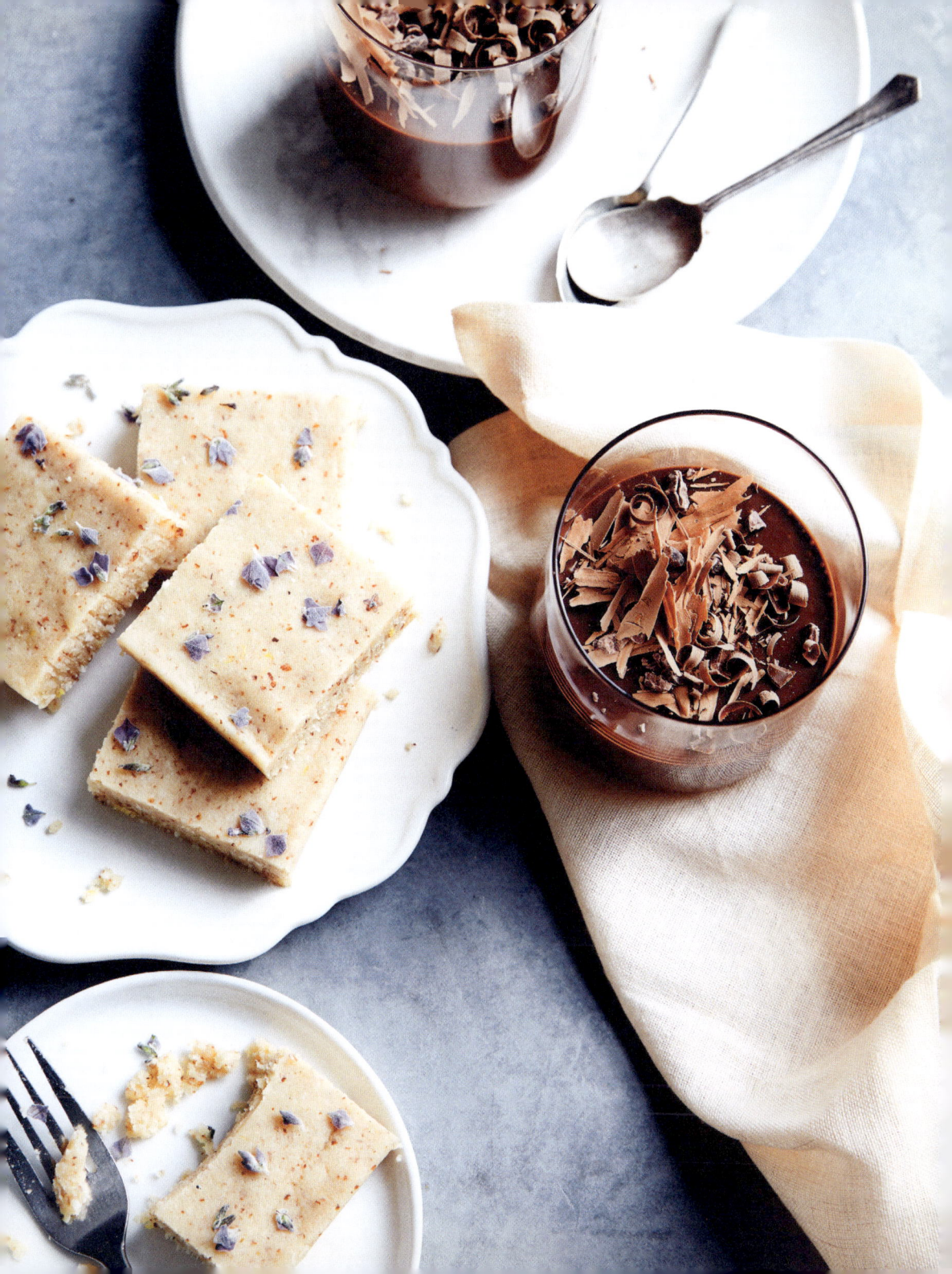

LEMON AND LAVENDER PROTEIN SLICE

Delicious treats at the ready help you to keep away from sugar-laden processed foods. This certainly is one delectable treat!

1 ½ cups almond meal

½ cup desiccated coconut

3 heaped tablespoons protein powder

3 tablespoons pure maple syrup

juice of 1 lemon

zest of 1 lemon

½ cup coconut oil, melted

pinch of pink salt

2 lavender sprigs

MAKES ONE BAKING TRAY

1. Place all ingredients, except lavender, in your food processor and blitz on high for 30 seconds.

2. Place the mixture into a tin lined with baking paper and press it down firmly. Sprinkle with lavender.

3. Pop it in the fridge and leave for around 60 minutes, or until firm.

4. Cut up into bite-sized slices. Store in an airtight container in the fridge or freezer.

Tip: If you don't have any fresh lavender, this is just as delicious without it.

BLISS BALLS

Medjool dates are a type of date which, though dried, are still soft and moist. They are sold loose or packaged. If you can't find medjool dates, the recipe will also work well with normal dates from the supermarket.

1 ½ cups almonds

1 cup medjool dates (seeds removed)

½ cup cacao butter

1 cup shredded coconut

1 tablespoon honey

½ cup protein powder

3 tablespoons cacao

1 tablespoon chia seeds

MAKES ABOUT 15

1. Simply whiz all ingredients together in a food processor until well processed and combined. You want it to be a nice consistency that you can roll together and make small balls. If it needs more moisture, simply add a tablespoon of water until it is the right consistency.

2. Store in the fridge in an airtight container.

HUMMUS AND VEGGIE SNACKS

Makes one generous bowl of hummus. Store-bought hummus can be
a wonderful snack when you feel the need for speed. But if you
wish to make your own, here's my favourite recipe.

400 g (14 oz) can
chickpeas, drained

1 cup water

2 tablespoons tahini

2-3 tablespoons virgin
olive oil

juice of 1 lemon

salt and pepper, to taste

vegetables, cut into
sticks, to serve

crackers, to serve

SERVES 4

1. Place all hummus ingredients in a food processor
   and whiz on high for approximately 15-20 seconds.
   Scrape down sides and check consistency. It should
   begin to resemble a smooth dip. Add more water if
   necessary.

2. Transfer to a sealed container and refrigerate. It will
   last in the fridge for 2-3 days.

3. Eat with carrot, cucumber or celery sticks or your
   favourite rice or gluten-free crackers.

BANANA NICE-CREAM

Could a recipe be any easier? This is wonderful for those summer evenings when you feel like a treat! You'll need to prepare the bananas for this recipe ahead of time. I like to have bananas in the freezer always. I cut them in half and store them in glad bags when they look like they are getting too ripe.

1 frozen banana

1 teaspoon cacao

3-5 ice cubes

SERVES 1

1. Combine in food processor and whiz on high until consistency resembles ice-cream.

2. Serve immediately.

Tip: You may be adventurous with this recipe (like all of my recipes) and add or substitute cacao for berries, mango or any fruit you wish. You can prepare and freeze these as well but the mixture will need to be whizzed again before serving.

LAYERED CARAMEL SLICE

Once you have all your ingredients set out, this slice is very simple to make. Loving Earth Caramel Luvju bars are my favourite brand of raw chocolate, but you can use whatever works for you. If you can't find it at your supermarket or grocer, use any good quality block of dark chocolate.

BOTTOM LAYER

1 cup almonds

1 tablespoon coconut oil

1 teaspoon cacao

3 tablespoons coconut nectar or honey

MIDDLE LAYER

½ cup peanut butter

¼ cup hazelnuts

2 tablespoons tahini

½ cup honey (or for low fructose, use either rice malt syrup or coconut nectar)

pinch of salt

pinch of vanilla bean powder (or vanilla essence)

TOP LAYER

1 cup macadamias

1 teaspoon coconut oil

2 teaspoons coconut flour

pinch of salt

4 tablespoons rice malt syrup

ICED LAYER

1 block of Loving Earth Caramel Luvju or 30 g (1 oz) raw chocolate (or chocolate of your choice)

raspberries, to garnish

SERVES 10

1. Line a bread tin or similar sized tin (this makes around 10 long slices) with baking paper.

2. To make the bottom layer, place all bottom layer ingredients in a food processor and chop until it resembles breadcrumbs. You may need to add a little water (and when I say a little, I mean a little - add a teaspoon at a time). Once well mixed, press into the bottom of the tin.

3. Repeat the same process for the middle layer and top layer.

4. For the iced layer, melt the chocolate and pour over the other layers. Allow to set for about 5 minutes. (Score the slice pieces before the chocolate fully sets so it cuts nicely.) Arrange raspberries on top.

5. Place in the refrigerator and take out just before serving.

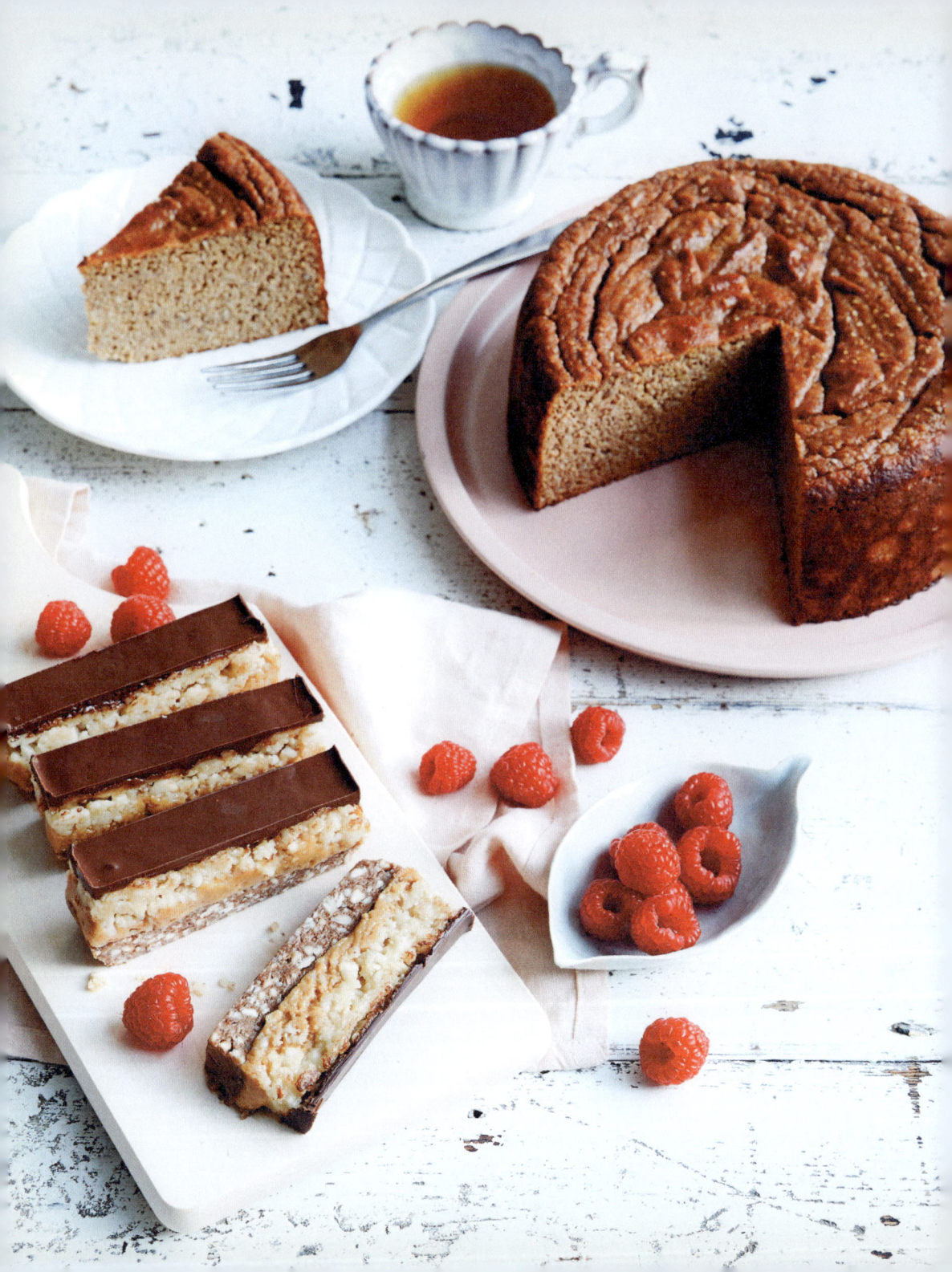

ORANGE AND CHOC CHIA SEED CAKE

This cake takes a while to cook, but is so worth it. In fact, I've been known to eat it for breakfast! Rice malt syrup is fructose free and available at all good supermarkets.

2 oranges, tops removed, cut and scored with a cross about 3 cm deep

6 organic free-range eggs

100 g (3 oz) rice malt syrup

250 g (8 oz) almond meal

2 tablespoons cacao

3 teaspoons baking powder

2 tablespoons soaked chia seeds

SERVES 12

1. Place the prepared oranges in a medium saucepan and cover with water. Bring to the boil and simmer for 50 minutes. Remove from the water and purée the whole orange, including peel, in a food processor until smooth.

2. Preheat oven to 160°C (320°F).

3. In a large mixing bowl, mix the eggs and rice malt syrup until light and fluffy. Add the almond meal, cacao and baking powder. Mix until combined. Stir in the orange purée and soaked chia seeds. Pour the mixture into a 22 cm cake tin lined with greaseproof baking paper. Do not use foil.

4. Bake in the oven for 40 minutes or until firm, but still moist. It may need to cook for up to 50 minutes. Leave to cool in the tin for about 5 minutes, then turn onto a wire rack and cool there.

Dinner

Simplicity is key for me as a multitasking modern day gal. Here are a bunch of my favourite 'easy as ABC' recipes that will stop you overloading on fast food. Each are 1–2 serves and can be kept in the fridge for leftovers to take with you the next day. You'll find most are gluten, dairy and refined sugar free – I've done the hard work for you, now it's your turn to simply prepare and enjoy.

ROAST CHICKEN

Roasting is one of the easiest ways to prepare succulent meat. Roast chicken is super easy to prepare and it is also an excellent source of collagen/gelatin which helps support good gut health. It can be used in the sushi bowl and yummo chicken salad recipes in this book.

1 organic or free-range chicken (whole)

2 –3 tablespoons olive oil

salt and pepper, to taste

SERVES 6

1. Preheat oven to 180°C (350°F).

2. Place chicken in a baking dish, drizzle with oil, and season with salt and pepper.

3. Place in oven and cook for approximately one hour, or until the juices run clear when you insert a knife next to the thigh.

Tip: You might like to roast some vegetables while you have your oven going to serve with the chicken.

SHIITAKE MUSHROOM SOUP

This recipe is comfort food at its best. Perfect as a winter warmer
to have you feeling fuller for longer with the added benefits of
pearl barley – high in fibre for balanced hormones.

8 dried shiitake
mushrooms (or
mushrooms of your
choice)

1 tablespoon oil
(preferably coconut oil)

4 spring onions, chopped

2 cloves garlic, crushed

1 celery stick, diced

1 carrot, diced

250 g (8 oz) fresh
shiitake mushrooms,
chopped

2 litres (8 cups)
vegetable stock

200 g (7 oz) pearl barley

SERVES 4

1. Place dried mushrooms in a bowl with hot water.
   Soak for 30 minutes. Once soaked, squeeze out the
   liquid from the mushrooms and slice thinly.

2. Heat oil in a pan over medium heat. Add spring
   onions, garlic, celery, carrot and fresh mushrooms.
   Cook for a few minutes, stirring, until softened.
   Add stock, barley and ½ cup water, and bring
   to the boil. Reduce heat and simmer for about
   40 minutes, until the barley is tender.

3. Plate up and enjoy!

YOU ARE WHAT YOU EAT

AROMATIC CHICKEN STOCK

I like to make fresh stock when making chicken soup. It can be frozen or kept in the fridge for a quick and easy addition to soups and stews.

1 organic or free-range chicken (whole)

3-4 litres (1 gallon) water, depending on the size of the chicken and pot

1 onion, cut into quarters

2 carrots, cut into quarters

1 zucchini, cut into quarters

2.5 cm (1 inch) piece fresh ginger, grated

2.5 cm (1 inch) piece fresh turmeric, grated

salt and pepper, to season (be generous, remember this is stock)

1. Place all ingredients in a large pot over medium heat and allow to simmer for 3-4 hours.

2. Once cooked, remove chicken and set aside (you will use this in your chicken soup following). Remove vegetables and discard (or eat if you like but they will be very soggy).

3. This stock can be frozen into batches or ice-cubes and used as needed. For the following soup you will need roughly 4 cups of stock.

4. Pull away the chicken meat for use in chicken soup.

CHICKEN SOUP

With the stock prepared, this soup is a quick, nutritious meal.

4 cups chicken stock

4 cups water

vegetables of your choice, such as 1 carrot, 2 sticks celery, 1 onion, chopped (optional)

chicken meat from 1 cooked chicken (from aromatic chicken stock)

250 g (8 oz) packet of rice or gluten-free noodles or noodles of your choice

goat's cheese, to serve

SERVES 4-6

1. Place stock in a pot and add 4 cups water.

2. If you choose to add vegetables, now is the time. You can add whatever your heart desires. My people love it when it is just chicken noodle, but I switch it up from time to time.

3. Place chicken meat in the soup. Add noodles and simmer over medium heat until cooked.

4. Serve with shavings of hard goat's cheese or eat as is!

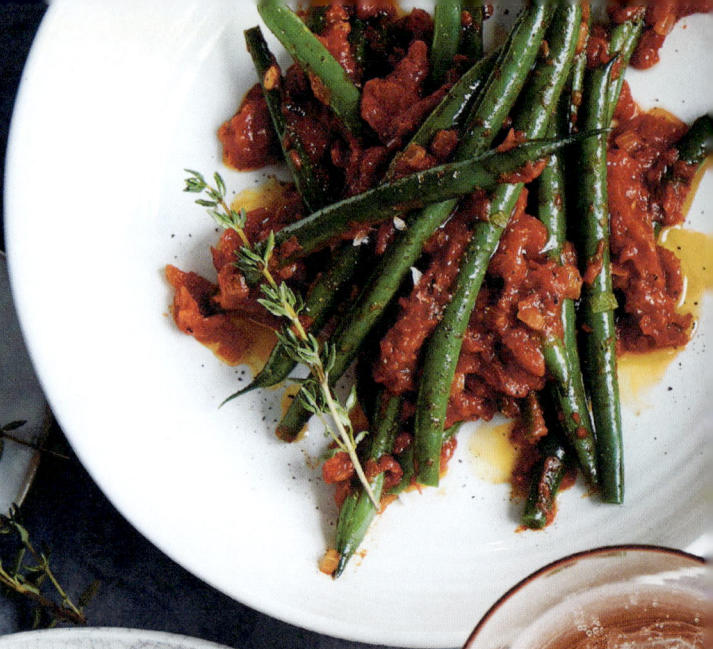

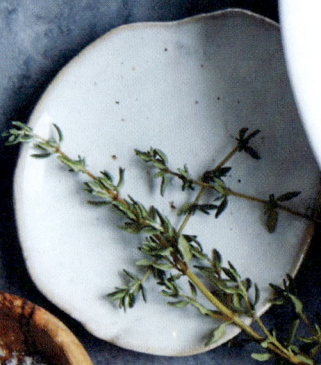

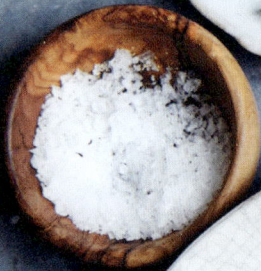

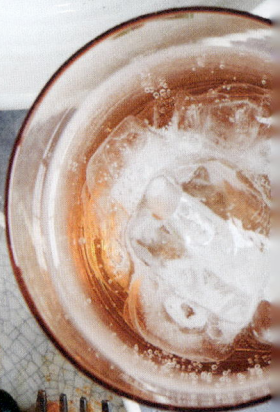

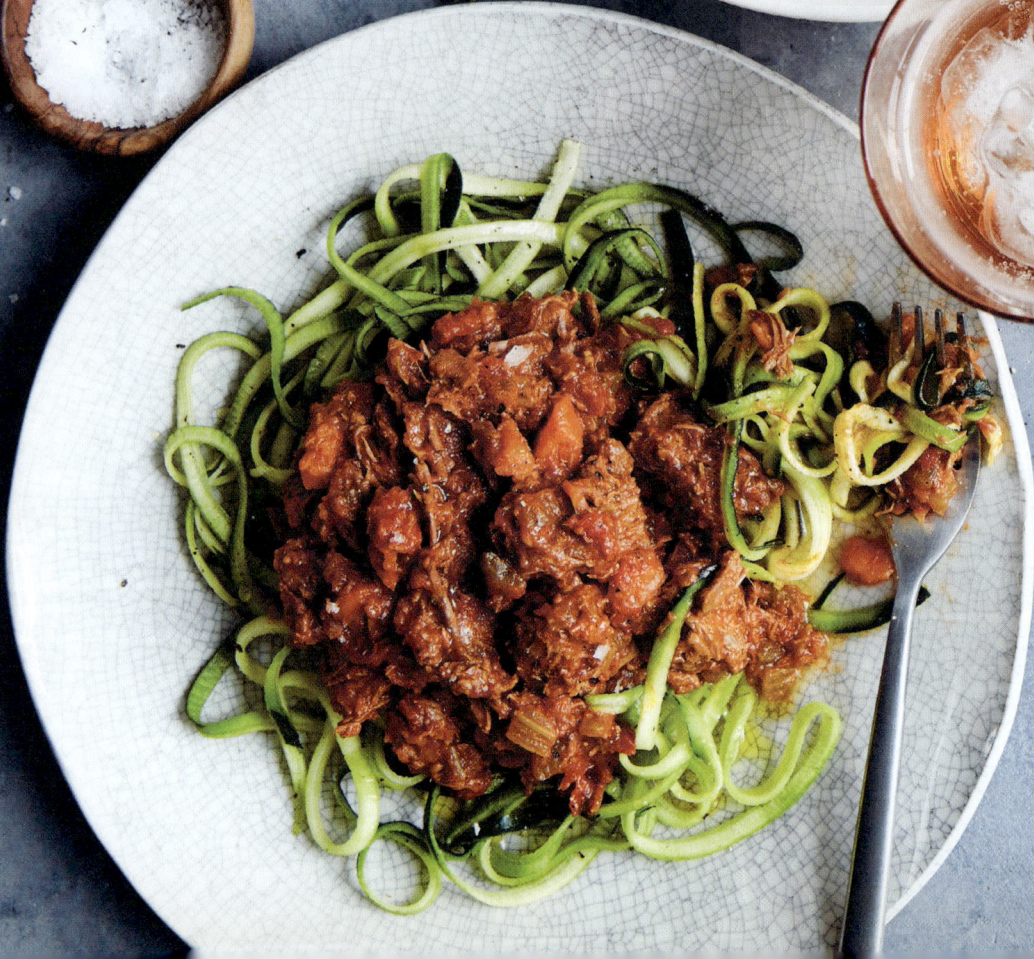

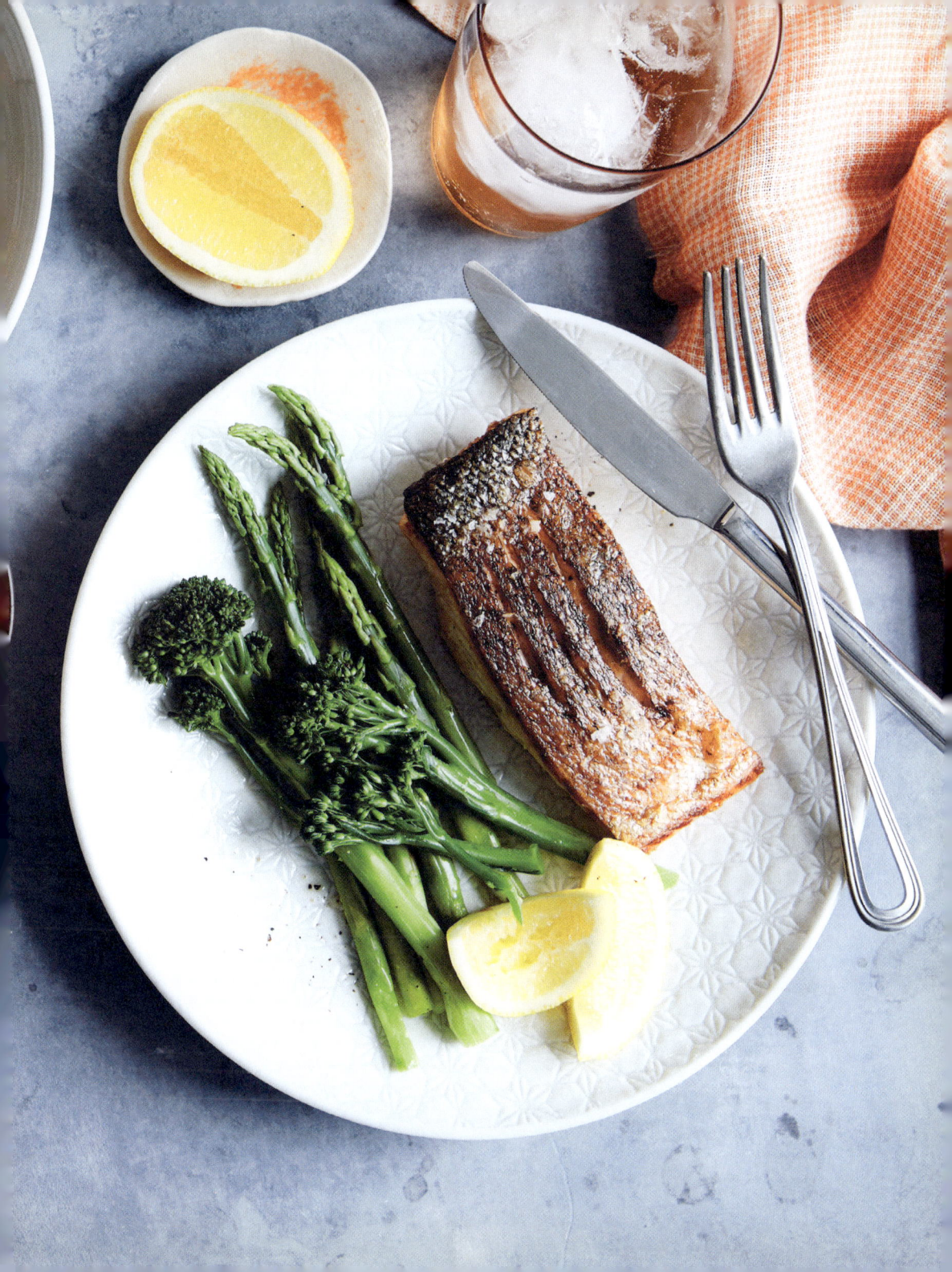

BAKED SALMON WITH ASPARAGUS AND BROCCOLINI

I would eat salmon every day of the week if my people let me! It's an excellent source of both fat and protein, and can be enjoyed in a variety of ways. Cooking it in the oven is super easy. Varieties of broccoli are excellent for oestrogen clearing. Including them in the diet regularly can be an easy addition to keep your hormones happier. Asparagus is also a prebiotic, excellent to feed the good gut bacteria.

2 pieces of salmon, skin on optional (I prefer the skin still on)

juice of 1 lemon

2–3 tablespoons olive oil

salt and pepper, to taste

1 bunch asparagus

1 bunch broccolini

extra olive oil for vegetables

SERVES 2

1. Preheat oven to 180°C (350°F).

2. Place salmon pieces in an oven dish. Pour lemon juice over the salmon and drizzle olive oil. Season as desired.

3. Place salmon in the oven and cook for approximately 20 minutes, or until it's cooked to your liking. I like salmon medium so the centre is still pink.

4. Meanwhile, place a double-boiler steamer on the stove. Add asparagus and broccolini, and steam until cooked. Place asparagus and broccolini in a bowl and drizzle with extra oil, season with salt and pepper and serve alongside salmon.

SLOW-COOKED BEEF RAGU WITH SPIRALISED ZUCCHINI

Slow-cooked meats are not only amazing for your gut but equally simple to digest, helping you overcome bloating, too. This recipe also happens to be completely delicious.

2 tablespoons oil

500 g (1 lb) chuck steak

1 onion, diced

2 sticks celery, chopped

1 carrot, chopped

1 can organic tomatoes

2 cups water or stock/broth

salt and pepper, to taste

2 zucchini, for spiralising

SERVES 2

1. Heat oil in a large heavy-based pan. Make sure the pan is hot, then sear the chuck steak on each side until browned (about 2–3 minutes).

2. Remove and set aside.

3. Turn heat down to medium; add onion and fry until clear.

4. Add celery and carrot, and sauté for about 3 minutes.

5. Add tomatoes and water or stock, season with salt and pepper. Return the meat to the pan. Turn heat down to low. Cover and cook for 2.5 hours, or until meat is tender and easy to break apart.

6. When ready to serve, spiralise zucchini. You can cook it if you wish, but I prefer it raw. Place spiralised zucchini in a bowl and top with ragu.

BRAISED BEANS WITH TOMATO

This is a stand-alone dish or you could serve it with protein of your choice.
It is a delicious vegetarian option which includes the wonderful antibacterial
and prebiotic benefits of garlic, plus the warming qualities of ginger.

2 tablespoons olive oil

2 onions, chopped

2 cloves garlic, finely chopped or crushed

3 teaspoons grated ginger

400 g (14 oz) can tomatoes

10 thyme sprigs

3 tablespoons red wine vinegar

300 g (10 oz) green beans, ends trimmed off

SERVES 4

1. Preheat oven to 160°C (320°F).

2. Place olive oil in an ovenproof pan over high heat on the stove (if you do not have an ovenproof pan, you will need to use two separate dishes).

3. Add onion, garlic and ginger and sweat until translucent - about 5 minutes.

4. Add tomatoes and thyme, and cook for a few minutes before adding vinegar. Bring to a simmer.

5. Place baking paper over the pan and cover with foil. Transfer to oven and roast for 1-1.5 hours (or as long as possible really - up to 4 hours; it gets more delicious as time goes on).

6. Increase oven temperature to 180°C (350°F) and place beans in the pan. Recover with baking paper and foil and roast for a further 20 minutes, or until beans are cooked.

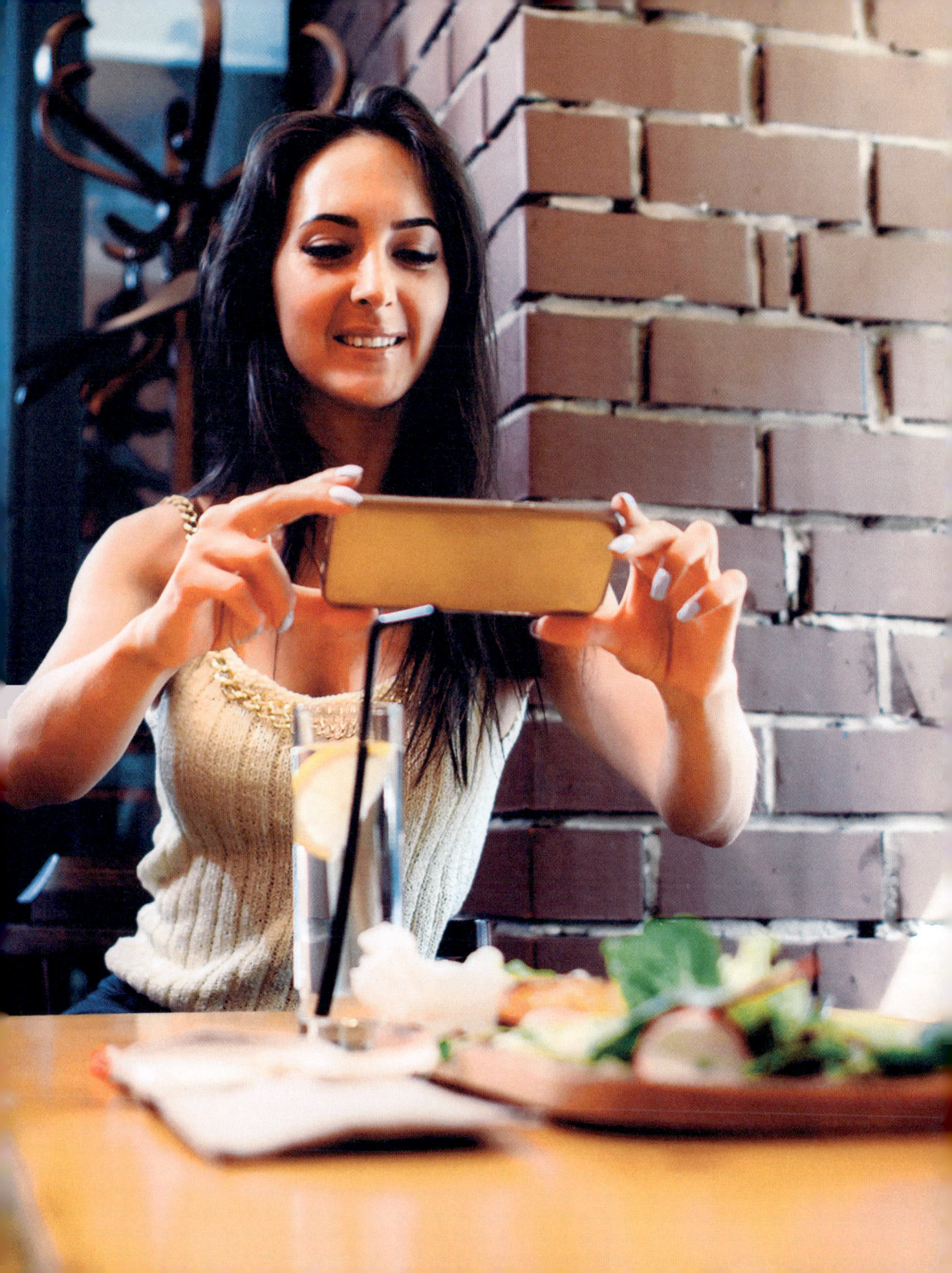

CHAPTER 11

Your affirmations

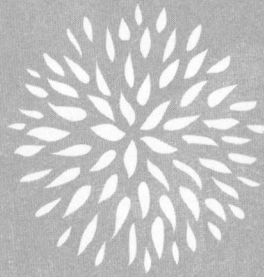

Worry is like praying for the exact thing you don't actually want.

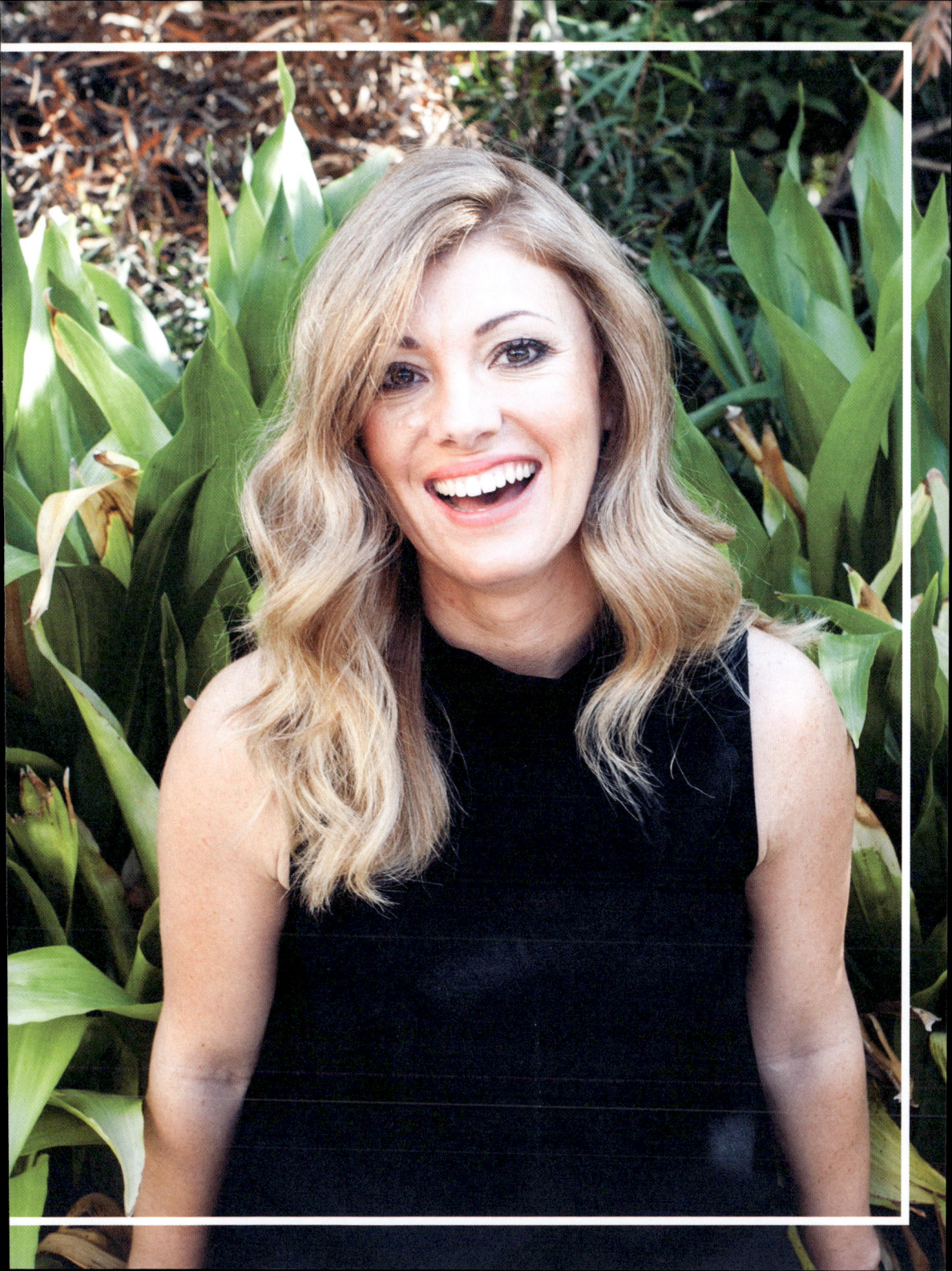

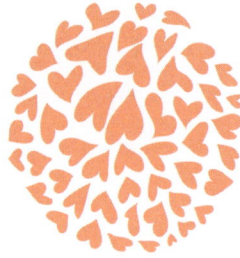

You're a boss

YOU WILL LEARN:

• what affirmations are and how they help

• how to make your own affirmations

Affirmations are extremely powerful additions to your life; in fact, consider them your superpower or secret weapon to tap into what you want. From a really early age, we are conditioned to feed the fears – it's human nature. We've gotten so good at focusing on exactly what we don't want, whether we worry about it, think about it or have it in the back of our mind, it still all adds to the 'don't want' pile. This is what may be better known as worry. Worry is like praying for the exact thing you don't actually want.

For me, affirmations have become a powerful game-changer. I see them as my very own slipstream towards activating and achieving exactly what I would like to happen in my life. Now of course, sometimes it may take a little while to get there and things don't necessarily work to immediate plan; however, operating out of this space of positivity certainly does change your perspective on life. My motto is always act as if any challenge or issue was placed in front of me to help me get what I want. Once I started operating from this mindset, my entire life changed.

> Affirmations may also be referred to as mantras, confirmations, declarations, statements – whatever resonates with you; they are, after all, your own set of powerful words that proclaim exactly what you want out of life.

Perhaps you've got a problem you can't see a way out of or maybe you have big hopes and dreams you're keen to activate. This is where your affirmations become your director, to keep you focused on the good and aligned to helping you continue to create more greatness in your life. It doesn't mean your mind at times doesn't wander to the negative; in fact, it's when your mind does go off course and start focusing on all the 'don't wants' that your mantra comes into play. **When you find yourself having your own pity party, this is when your mantra is most powerful.**

How to create your mantra

Ask yourself, do I have a problem or am I wanting to make something happen in my life? Or is there an ache in the pit of your stomach that seems to always be there even when you're having a good day? Whatever you choose isn't wrong, you can use your affirmation for whatever you need. In fact, you might have several that you use at once (guilty).

I like to outline my mantra and then save it in my phone to pop up at a certain time each day. It's common for me to have at least two, maybe even three that appear at specific times – usually around 11 am, 1 pm and again at 3 pm. This helps keep me motivated and in check, and if I'm having a particularly testing or troublesome day (or a pity party), it can help remind me that life is generally fabulous and it's all there for me – all I need to do is choose.

HERE'S HOW - IF I HAVE A PROBLEM

I. I like to flip things around and ask myself, 'What if this problem was put here to help me get exactly what I wanted?'

2. I then say to myself, 'If I could make the solution of this problem be anything I wanted, what would that be? What would be my ultimate outcome?'

3. I then begin to imagine my out-of-this-world, crazy, beautiful ultimate outcome. Almost as if it were a movie, I watch it play out in my mind, all the while continuing to ask myself, 'If this was my ultimate outcome, how would it make me feel?' Perhaps it may make me feel happy, relieved, exhilarated, accomplished … whatever that is for you.

Whenever the problem pops back into my mind, I remind myself of this feeling (happy, relieved, exhilarated, accomplished, etc.) to switch back over to where I'm headed. From this I then create my affirmation, for example:

*'Today I feel happy because I am always
able to create my reality.'*

Now it's your turn: (fill in the blanks)

1. PROBLEM

2. IDEAL SOLUTION

3. WORDS THAT EXPLAIN HOW I FEEL WITH THE
   PERFECT/IDEAL SOLUTION

HERE'S HOW - IF I WANT TO ACHIEVE SOMETHING

Phase 1 - Celebrate the wins

I. Make a list of the top three things you've achieved in the last year. It may be a grade, an achievement or a goal that you kicked butt in doing.

2. Explain how you made each one come to life. Examples might be: enrolled into a course and worked the summer to pay the fees; or gave myself permission to study really hard at all costs. Whatever it is, there is no right or wrong.

3. Find a sentence about the underlying belief that took you to achieve your goal. Maybe it was driven by the feeling of relief once it was done or the fact that you gained something when the achievement had been ticked off. What drove you to finish?

Once you have outlined this you can see how you've achieved something you wanted, possibly without a conscious mantra but with a purpose, reason and method. A mantra is how you cement this method for your next achievement, consciously. Now you can see how you've achieved your top three things from the past year, it's time to make new ones come to the forefront of your mind.

But before you do - see these three achievements you've made happen? You must know how powerful you are as the creator of your life. YOU made these things happen all because you are beautifully you, an incredible and capable human being with the will to do whatever you so desire.

Perhaps you know somebody who has the wildest spirit. Like really crazy but they seem to just have life land in their lap. They name what they want and they get it, as it if is almost effortless. They have tapped into this slipstream, whether they realise it or not. And while their dreams seem totally insane to you, they achieve them.

Remember – what we focus on, expands.

Now we've told ourselves we are so amazing and awesome we can replicate this affirmation, not from looking where we've come from, but where we now want to go. What powerful motivation!

Phase 2 - Create your own mantra

You can have as many of these going at once as you like, but to really drill down and get your mantra or affirmation, let's go with one thing. What's one thing you want to achieve this year?

I. Identify your goal. What is it that you want to achieve? Maybe it's to have a best friend who understands you completely or that you want to ace your biology exam or that you want to do well in a job interview or presentation. Whatever it is, write it down.

2. How would it make you feel if you achieved it? Write down three words to describe this feeling. Maybe it's relieved, supported and happy. Use a thesaurus to assist if needed to really get some juicy words to help you.

3. Now use these words, speaking in the present tense (not past or future because what you are wanting to create, while it is in the future, starts now).

The biggest whoopsie we can make is making all of our goals for the future or someday. Your someday starts now.

Your affirmation comes directly from this. Here are some examples.

'I feel relieved and happy knowing that my biology exam is in the bag because I am supported and able.'

'My biology exam is in the bag and I feel happy, supported and relieved.'

It can be whatever you want it to be, so long as you ensure the following:

- Your affirmation is YOUR affirmation – not somebody else's.
- It contains the words 'I' or 'my'.
- It's spoken as if it is happening no matter what – there is no maybe about it.
- It's happening now – in real time.

Have you ever watched your friend or somebody you follow on Instagram LIVE but not in real time? It's nowhere near as fun as in real time. Your affirmation is no different. It's happening in real time – remember that!

Now it's your turn.

List the top three things you've achieved this year.

Explain how you made them happen.

Create a sentence that helps you achieve each of these.

Celebrate YOU.

Now create your own affirmation.

List your goal.

List three words that describe how you would feel if you were
to achieve this goal.

Now create your affirmation.

Remember to pop these affirmations somewhere you can see them regularly and check back in. Your affirmations, while useful when you feel like you're on fire and kicking goals in life, become even more powerful when you can tap into using them to switch the station when things aren't seeming to work out for you. We can easily get bogged down by the crappy things that happen, or we focus on all the good that seems to happen to everybody else and feel like we're missing out. Truth is, you hold the remote.

When you find yourself down and out, first up is recognising this feeling and that it may pass in 90 seconds, and second to this is choosing again. Often when we are feeling this, we are in a parasympathetic state; that is, we are on auto stress mode or, as I like to refer to it with my patients, battle mode. Being in battle mode can save your life, but we can't remain in this state for long periods of time. It becomes our undoing. When you find yourself in fight or flight with the negative soundtrack on repeat, here's how to get yourself out.

1. Grab your affirmation. Close your eyes.
2. Take 5 large breaths right down into your abdomen, breathing in for 5 and out for 5.
3. Start to play your mind movie of how you want your goal to play out and remember how this makes you feel when you achieve it.
4. Repeat your affirmation (you guessed it) 5 times.

With all this growing and changing, it's important to remember that your body knows what to do and will do it at the right time for you. Throughout your teens and through to your late 20s, you will continue to grow and change shape. Remember that you will grow on your own schedule and you will have your own unique vibe. Do your best to trust your body and take care of it so it can help you accomplish lots of great things.

Getting down to business – your 3-month program

Learning about your menstrual cycle doesn't have to be tricky. In fact, it can be the freedom you're searching for, since your body is dishing up to you information about the internal state of your body in every second of every day.

Every day we experience highs, lows and everything in between. This diary will help you understand your body better, and watch the ebbs and flows of your hormones and the rhythms that they bring. Use the icons and fill in each day to reflect how you feel as well as map what your body is telling you. For example, on Monday, if you have your period and you feel tired, you'd fill in with the ⚋ and ✖ icons. Over time you can learn to predict and understand your signs and symptoms.

There is a sample page below, to show you what I mean. Then go ahead and use the pages that follow to create your diary.

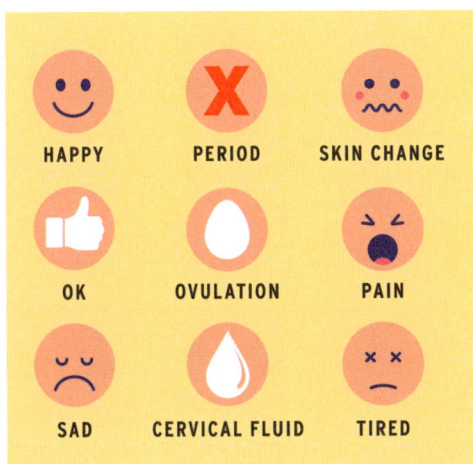

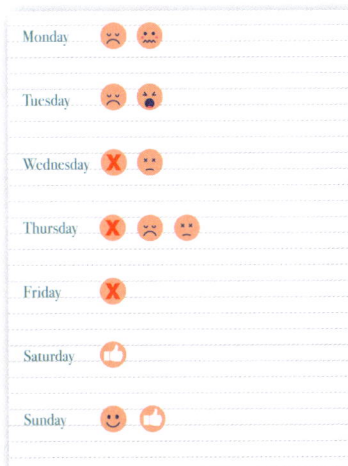

HAPPY	PERIOD	SKIN CHANGE
OK	OVULATION	PAIN
SAD	CERVICAL FLUID	TIRED

Monday	
Tuesday	
Wednesday	
Thursday	
Friday	
Saturday	
Sunday	

Monday

Tuesday

Wednesday

Thursday

Friday

Saturday

Sunday

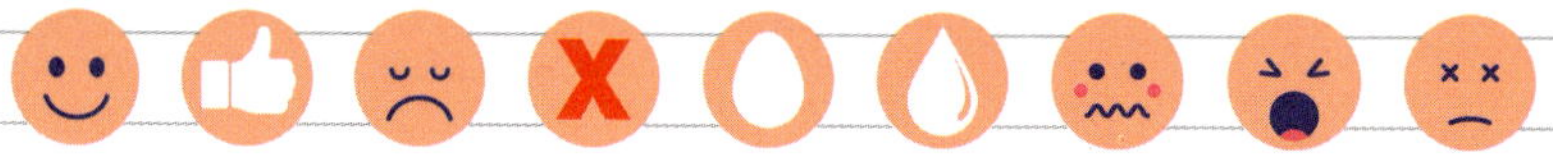

Monday

Tuesday

Wednesday

Thursday

Friday

Saturday

Sunday

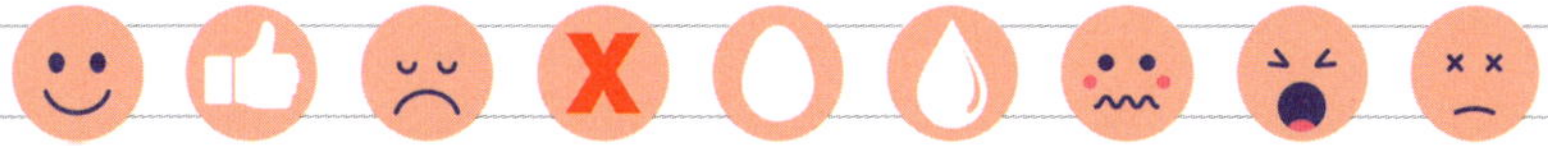

Monday

Tuesday

Wednesday

Thursday

Friday

Saturday

Sunday

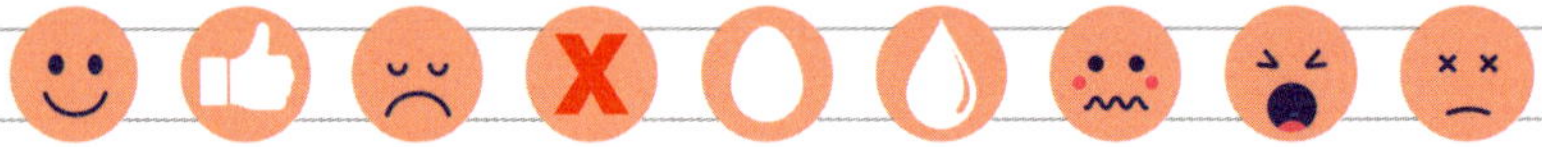

Monday

Tuesday

Wednesday

Thursday

Friday

Saturday

Sunday

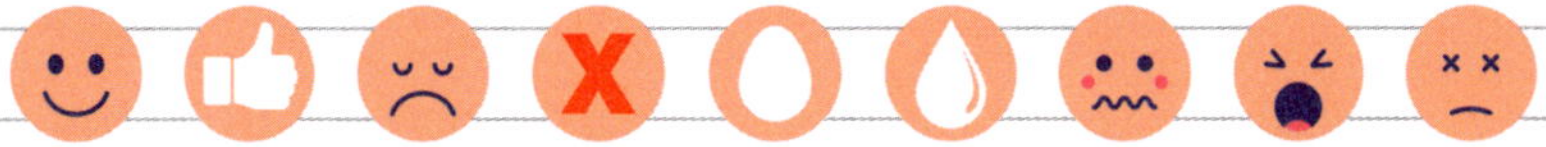

Monday

Tuesday

Wednesday

Thursday

Friday

Saturday

Sunday

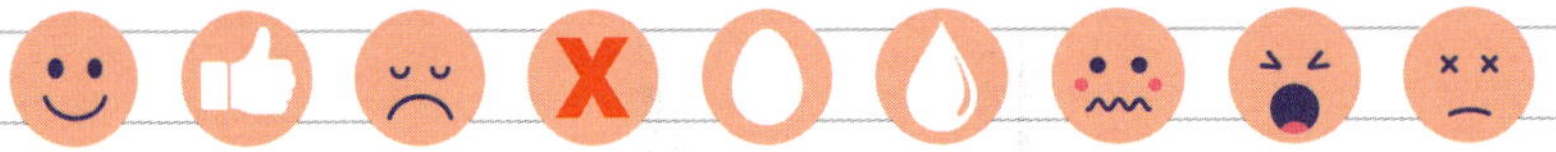

Monday

Tuesday

Wednesday

Thursday

Friday

Saturday

Sunday

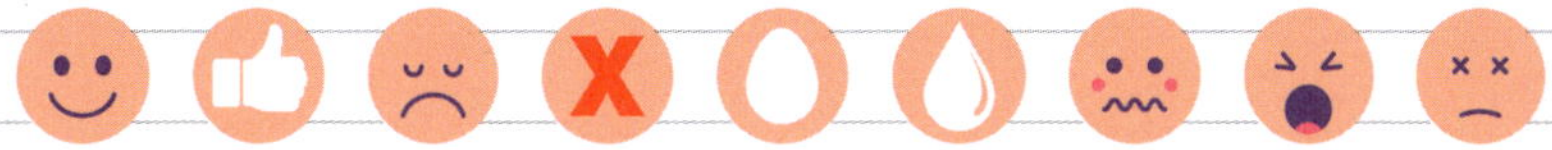

Monday

Tuesday

Wednesday

Thursday

Friday

Saturday

Sunday

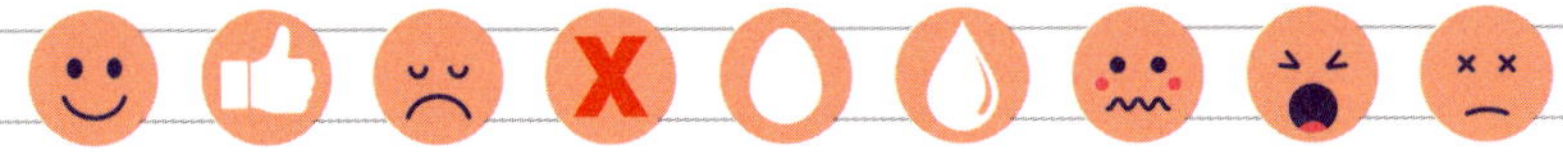

Monday

Tuesday

Wednesday

Thursday

Friday

Saturday

Sunday

Monday

Tuesday

Wednesday

Thursday

Friday

Saturday

Sunday

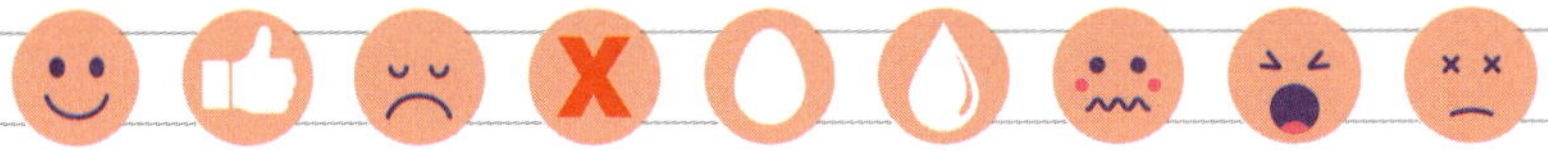

Monday

Tuesday

Wednesday

Thursday

Friday

Saturday

Sunday

Monday

Tuesday

Wednesday

Thursday

Friday

Saturday

Sunday

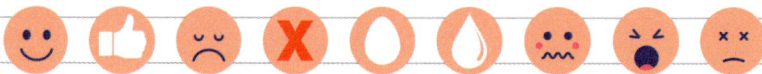

Monday

Tuesday

Wednesday

Thursday

Friday

Saturday

Sunday

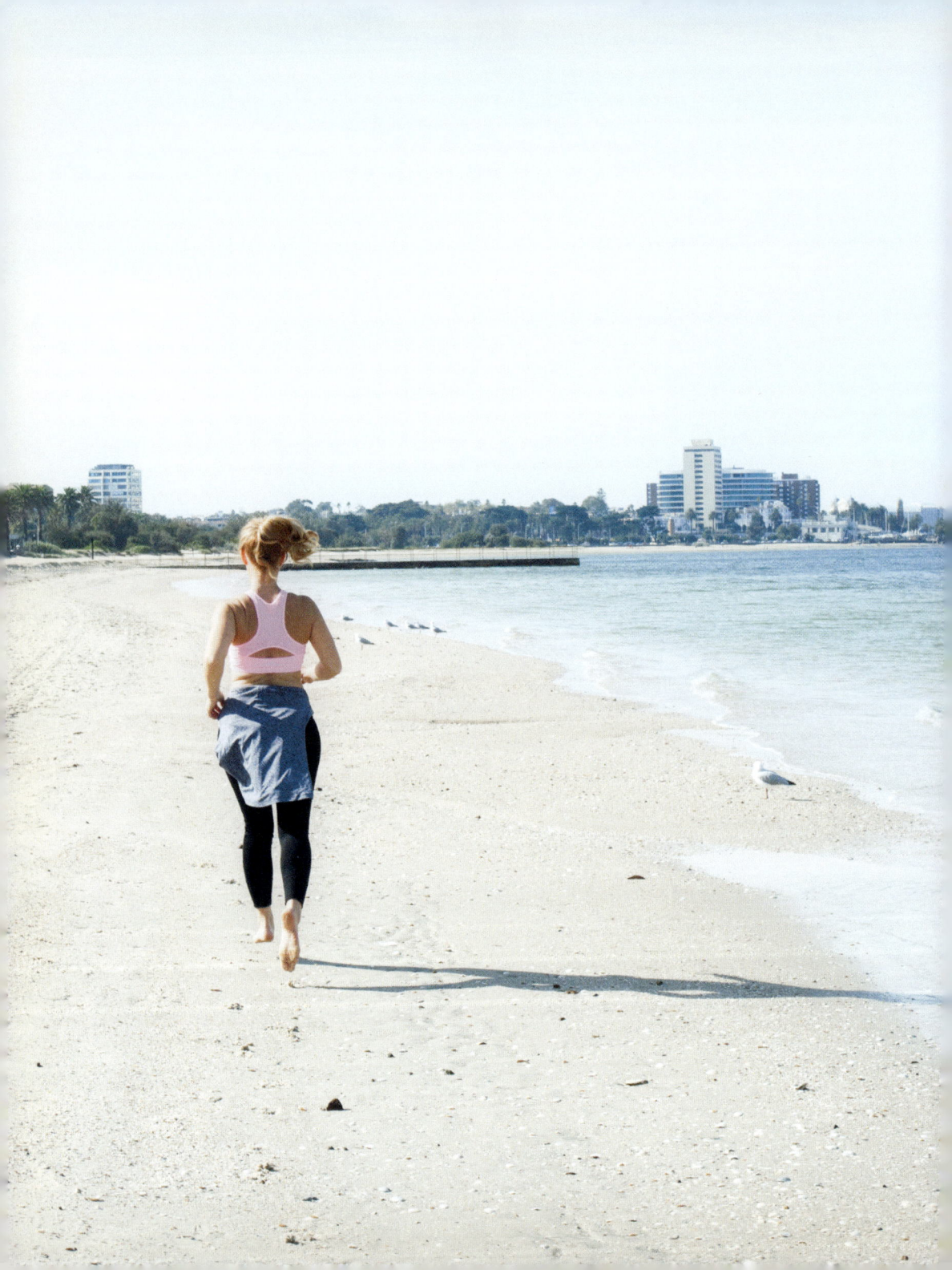

How do I even begin to say thank you …

There has been an abundance of people in my life who have supported me in my ongoing path as a healthcare practitioner and to you I want to say thank you. It's difficult to know where to start.

First up, I'm so grateful for you, my reader. As a woman, I'm so proud of you for taking the time to get to know your body that much better and whether you're a mama reading this book to pass on to your precious daughter or the daughter absorbing this information, know that you are already out of the category of 'average woman' all because you're so keen to learn more about yourself and your body. Accepting that we are all different and always learning is just so beautiful. You as a woman inspire me each and every day to give back, to continue to be a voice among women and to lead from this feminine and divine space. I love us. We've got this.

My incredible husband – while I may be a total brat at times, you continue to support me each and every day and nothing I ever say is too crazy or impossible. You let me be me and for that I love you dearly. Thank you for being the yin to my yang and for your constant unconditional love and support. I love doing life with you. I do ultimately love your insta stories (even if they are on my Instagram!). Most of all, thank you for choosing me to be the mama of our children and to inspire them to be everything they will become.

To Olivia and Geordie, my babies. My oh my, you guys are quite the daily self check-in that I need consistently. Thank you for choosing me and for allowing me to continue to learn and grow because of you. I know you were both sent our way for a reason. I love you both so very much and am so proud of you both.

My own mum and dad, for being my biggest fans, for showing me that anything is possible, and for loving me just as I am. I'm a very lucky girl. I still remember the day I said to Mum, 'I'll be famous someday, not because I want fame, but because I really want to make a massive difference in people's lives.' And I still remember your answer, Mum, 'Yup Nat, I know.' Thank you both, you are the perfect example of what parents should be. You are both amazing.

My sister Hollie and her beautiful family, for the ongoing love and support and constant words of encouragement. She may be taller, I feel I'm wiser – just by 4 years, even if people can't see it. I love you all beyond measure.

My mother-in-law Ouraina is a gift – she may not say much but I'd be totally lost without her love and care. My children are so fortunate to be able to have you around the corner (not to mention it helps me immensely!). Thank you for being our very own childcare centre and fast food outlet.

To my wingwoman and PA 'Amy' and my team, Erin, Alissa, Hannah, Wendy, Caleb, Sarah, Rachael, Jacinta, Maryanne and Bek. You guys seriously have no idea how proud and privileged I feel to work with you each day. We really are a dream team. Thank you for allowing me to create a space for us all to learn and grow.

I cannot put into words my respect and gratitude to Dr Shawn Tassone but I'll try. Thank you so very much for supporting me through this entire process, your input to the book, for reading it, correcting any silly mistakes and for questioning me on e v e r y t h i n g. Thanks for allowing me to argue physiology with you and for quickly becoming somebody I admire, and for the wonderful work you do for women worldwide. It most certainly doesn't go unnoticed. I feel very blessed to have you in my corner. Remember, your weaknesses are your strengths.

To my favourite gal pals – there's a long list – I want to make special mention of you. Each of you play a part in me being me, being my cheer squad, my therapy and my support network. I love you dearly. Aine – you always know what to say. Melina – we couldn't have been through more and managed to come out the other side (we're amazing). Fay – for just being raw and keeping me real. Sammy G – for the laughs and love about the biz. Chrissy – for always being there, always. Bec, my other wing woman – we do love ourselves so enough and we're worth it. Susanna, Alison, Lisa and the other school mamas – your support and checking in doesn't go unnoticed. Thank you for being my tribe.

To friends who get it because they live it too, I feel like I've known a lifetime. Lola, Cecelia, Tanya, my favourite Period Fixer, Nicole – I love you all; know that a part of this book comes from a part of you and our friendship. You inspire me.

Sarah Wagner, you are a darn legend. Thank you for seeing the bigger picture and for listening to my copious calls. Five years and counting as my agent and manager is a milestone in itself.

To my teachers and mentors, the Mindshare Mastermind group, JJ and Karl. I'm so grateful for your support, guidance and acceptance. You continue to blow my mind and to remind me to show up every day and serve others. Thank you.

To everybody else who has supported me in this journey, amazing publishers who saw the bigger picture, this wouldn't have happened without you. I feel completely blessed by it all.

Index

A

acne 12, 97–104
    hormone imbalance and 99
    menstrual cycle and 100
    the pill and 218–19
    treatment 101–3
acupuncture 58
adenomyosis 135
adrenaline 28
affirmations 274–6
    mantra, create your own
        276–80
allergies 81
amenorrhea 141–5
anatomy, our 196–206
    reproductive system 200–7
anovulatory bleeding 36
antibiotics 121–2
anus and rectum 200
attitude 55
autoimmunity 150–1

B

bloating 112–15
blue light 88
breast
    cancer 77
    changes 116
    formation, stages 117

C

cervix 197–8
    cervical fluid 36–7, 216–17
    Cervical Screening Test 51
circadian rhythm 44
clitoris 203–4
collagen 160
conception 218
contraception 171–7

cervical cap and diaphragm
    176
condoms 177
copper IUD 175–5
depo provera (injection)
    173–4
Fertility Awareness Method
    220
implanon (birth control
    implant) 173
long-term use of the pill 215
mirena 174–5
the pill 171–2
pregnancy after injections
    215
cortisol 27

D

decisions, working through 71
detoxification 84–5
DHEA 28
diagnosis 165–7
diet
    4-week plan 230
    bad fats 231
    good fats 226–8
    junk food 225–6

E

electromagnetic fields exposure
    (EMFs) 88
emotions
    90-second rule 59
    associated organs and 57
    emotional wellbeing 84
    ill-health, manifesting as 61–3
    supplements for mood
        support 110
    mood swings and PMS 105

endocrine system 23
endometriosis 128–30
    conception and 216
    flow chart 133
    tips to tackle 132
environment 85
exercise 186–7

F

fallopian tubes 197
fats
    bad 231
    good 226–8
feelings
    90-second rule 59
fertilisation 37–8
Fertility Awareness Method 220
food see diet
    processed foods 76
    recipes see Recipe index

G

genes 91
    missing periods and 142–3
glands 23–4
growth hormone 29
gut feelings 68, 70
gut wellbeing 82–3, 155–60
    foods, helpful 160
    leaky gut 83, 155
    microbiome 82
    supplements 159–60

H

habits, developing good 233
hair, pubic and underarm 118
herbs, to treat UTIs 123
hormone imbalance
    acne and 99

causes of 81–8
missing periods 141–2
symptoms 32
hormones see also hormone
   imbalance
   8-year cycles of hormones
      79
   adiponectin 30
   adrenaline 28
   cortisol 27
   DHEA 28
   growth 29
   insulin 28
   melanocyte-stimulating 29
   melatonin 28
   oestrogen 26
   progesterone 27
   role of 23, 26
   serotonin 29
   skin and 31
   testosterone 27
   thyroid hormones 29
   weight loss and 30, 31, 95–6
HPA axis 44
hypothalamus gland 23–4

I
immune system 23
infections, hidden 85–6
inflammation 149–51
   treatment 151
insulin resistance 152–4
   PCOS and 153
intolerances 81
intuition 68, 70

J
'The Journey' 61–3

L
leaky gut 83, 155
   foods 160

M
mantra, create your own 276–80
medications and missing
      periods 143
melanocyte-stimulating
      hormone 29
melatonin 28
menstrual cycle 44
   acne and 100
   late follicular phase 48
   luteal phase 49–50, 198
   'normal' 34
   ovulation stage 46–7
   post-menstrual/pre-
      ovulation 46
   premenstrual 47
   stages of, understanding
      44–8
metabolism 95, 96
microbiome 82
mindset 55
   observer effect 66–7
missing periods 141–5

N
nervous system 23
nutrient deficiencies 81–2

O
observer effect 66–7
oestrogen 26
   dietary 76
   estrobolome 83
   excess 77
orgasm 206–7

ovaries 196
ovulation 37–8, 46–7
   chart 39
   feeling 36
   irregular, early or late 38
   pain, dealing with 214

P
perimenopause 79
periods 33
   anovulatory bleeding 36
   cycle, 'normal' 34
   early onset of 76–7
   first, dread of 12
   missing 141–5
   pads or tampons 89
   pain 136–40, 212–13
   PMS see Premenstrual
      Syndrome (PMS)
   role of 33–4
   tampons, learning to use 12
pheromones 40
the pill 171–2, 218–19, 221
   acne and 218–19
   long-term use 215
pituitary gland 23–4
Polycystic Ovarian Syndrome
      (PCOS) 12, 27, 124–7
   diagnosis 124–5
   diet, best 214
   fertility and 216
   insulin and 153
   puberty and 97
   signs of 124
prebiotics 157
Premenstrual Syndrome
      (PMS) 23
   fixes 107–8
   mood swings and 105

supplements for mood
support 110
probiotic foods 82, 159
problems, an approach to 65
processed foods 76
progesterone 27, 38
puberty 97
stages of 117
pubic
hair 118
region 206

R
reproductive system 200–7
clitoris 203–4
orgasm 206–7
pubic region 206

S
serotonin 29
sex 208–9
sex hormone tests 51
sexually transmitted infections
(STIs) 86
skin 97–104
acne see acne
gut health and 97
hormones and 31
supplements 104
sleep 181–3
deprivation 182
socialising 188
friendships 190–1
soy 77
stress 54, 77, 184–5
poor response to 87
skin conditions and 101

where it manifests in body
59
sub-fertility 41
supplements
gut health 159–60
mood support 110
skin 104

T
tampons, learning to use 12
testing 169–70
testosterone 27, 98
thrush 217
thyroid 23–4, 29
Toxic Shock Syndrome (TSS) 89
toxin exposure 86–7
Traditional Chinese Medicine
(TCM) 56–7
8-year cycles of hormones
79
treatment, focus 60

U
urethra and bladder 200
urinary tract infections (UTIs)
121–3
herbal treatments 123
uterus 197

V
vagina 198
hymen 200
labia 199
odour 40, 118–19, 121
vaginal discharge 40
vulva 199

W
weight
factors determining 96
gain 95
hormones and 30, 31, 95–6

Z
zinc 160

Index of recipes

B

bananas
    fritter cakes 241
    nice-cream 257
beans, braised with tomato 270
beef ragu, slow-cooked with
spiralised zucchini 269
berries
    buckwheat berry pancakes
      242
    sweet strawberry parfait 240
bliss balls 255
breakfast
    almost omelette 238
    banana fritter cakes 241
    brekky bowl 236
    buckwheat berry pancakes
      242
    choc cherry chia pudding
      237
    sweet strawberry parfait 240
brekky bowl 236
buckwheat berry pancakes 242

C

cake, orange and choc chia
seed 261
caramel slice, layered 258
cherry chia pudding, choc 237
chia
    choc cherry chia pudding
      237
    orange and choc chia seed
cake 261
chicken
    roast 262
    soup 265
    stock 264
    yummy chicken salad 243
chocolate

choc cherry chia pudding
    237
mousse 252
orange and choc chia seed
    cake 261

D

dinner
    baked salmon with
      asparagus and broccolini
      268
    braised beans with tomato
      270
    chicken soup 265
    roast chicken 262
    shiitake mushroom soup 263
    slow-cooked beef ragu with
      spiralised zucchini 269

F

frittata, anytime 251

H

hummus and veggie snacks 256

L

lemon and lavender protein
    slice 254
lettuce cups 250
lunch
    anytime frittata 251
    chicken salad, yummo 243
    lettuce cups 250
    mish-mash lunch plate 246
    salad jar 247
    sushi bowl 248
    twisted zucchini lunch bowl
      249

O

omelette, almost 238
orange and choc chia seed
    cake 261

P

pancakes, buckwheat berry 242
parfait, sweet strawberry 240
protein slice, lemon and
    lavender 254

S

salads
    salad jar 247
    yummo chicken 243
salmon, baked with asparagus
    and broccolini 268
snacks and treats
    banana nice-cream 257
    bliss balls 255
    chocolate mousse 252
    hummus and veggie snacks
      256
    layered caramel slice 258
    lemon and lavender protein
      slice 254
    orange and choc chia seed
      cake 261
soup
    chicken 265
    shiitake mushroom 263
stock, chicken 264
sushi bowl 248

Z

zucchini
    slow-cooked beef ragu with
      spiralised zucchini 269
    twisted zucchini lunch bowl
      249

First published January 2019 by HQ Non Fiction
An imprint of Harlequin Enterprises (Australia) Pty Ltd.
Level 13, 201 Elizabeth St
SYDNEY NSW 2000
AUSTRALIA

ISBN 9781489256638

Cover design by Jane Waterhouse
Cover image by Chris Middleton
Internal design by Jane Waterhouse
All illustrations by Jane Waterhouse except vulvas by Robin Cowcher
Food styling by Deborah Kaloper
Home economist Sarah Watson
Photos of Nat on pages 10, 73, 93, 163, 193, 211, 223, 234 and food images on 158, 237, 244-245,
253, 260, 264-265 and 271 by Chris Middleton
Photos of Nat on pages 2, 19, 53, 147, 178, 273, 296 by Steph Brown Photography

Printed and bound in China by RR Donnelley